D1300329

Working with Divorcing Spouses

Working with Divorcing Spouses

How to Help Clients Navigate the Emotional and Legal Minefield

Sam Margulies

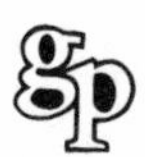

THE GUILFORD PRESS
New York London

Published by The Guilford Press
A Division of Guilford Publications, Inc.
72 Spring Street, New York, NY 10012
www.guilford.com

Printed in the United States of America

This book is printed on acid-free paper.

Last digit is print number: 9 8 7 6 5 4 3 2 1

Library of Congress Cataloging-in-Publication Data

Margulies, Sam.
Working with divorcing spouses : how to help clients navigate the emotional and legal minefield / by Sam Margulies.
p. ; cm.
Includes bibliographical references and index.
ISBN-13: 978-1-59385-481-2 (hardcover : alk. paper)
ISBN-10: 1-59385-481-1 (hardcover : alk. paper)
1. Divorce therapy. 2. Divorce mediation. 3. Divorce counseling. I. Title.
[DNLM: 1. Counseling–methods. 2. Divorce–psychology. 3. Divorce–legislation & jurisprudence. 4. Negotiating. 5. Psychotherapy–methods. WM 55 M331w 2007]
RC488.6.M37 2007
616.89′1562–dc22

2007010680

For Charles and Thelma Holloway

About the Author

Sam Margulies, PhD, JD, has been a pioneer in the field of mediation for 28 years. Instrumental in defining the field, he has taught mediation for 20 years, has made numerous presentations throughout the United States, and has published extensively. His book *Getting Divorced without Ruining Your Life* was one of the first to assert that divorce can be done decently, and without the devastation associated with traditional adversarial divorce. Dr. Margulies lives and practices mediation in Greensboro, North Carolina.

Preface

I have written this book to inform and embolden therapists who work with divorcing people. I am convinced that therapists, more than any other professional group, are best situated to improve the American way of divorce. Most divorces are preceded by a visit to a mental health professional by either or both members of a couple. In large numbers people turn to therapists to help them sort through their disappointment in their marriages and to guide them through the decision to divorce. It seems that, at least among the middle class, marriage counseling is perceived to be a necessary step prior to the decision to divorce. All this puts therapists in the ideal position to educate clients and guide them toward constructive rather than destructive divorce; the "good" divorce rather than the "bad." But the fact that therapists are positioned to help does not mean that many take the opportunity to do so. Either because they define it as beyond their proper therapeutic scope or because they fear treading on the turf of lawyers, most therapists stop short of guiding their clients through the divorce. It is that reluctance I want to address in this book. I want to provide therapists with the knowledge and understanding of divorce that will allow them to expand their role in the process of divorce. Much of what divorce lawyers do they do poorly because they are not trained to deal with emotions and relationship dynamics, which then results in untold damage to divorcing families. Therapists are the rightful occupiers of large pieces of turf that they have unwittingly and unnecessarily ceded to the legal profession. The purpose of this book is to get therapists to take back that turf.

After many years of practice in divorce law and mediation, I continue to be struck by how many people have unnecessarily bad divorces. Laypeople are woefully uninformed about divorce law and practice, including the subculture of lawyers, which generally promotes competitive adversarial behavior at the expense of collaborative and cooperative behavior. The public perception of such things is driven more by myth than fact, so that people on the cusp of divorce are vulnerable to information that directs them down often destructive paths. Most people are also unprepared for the emotional toll divorce can take, particularly during the early stages of the divorce. Feelings of fear, guilt, rejection, or humiliation easily provoke behavior that makes matters worse rather than better. Ignorance about the emotional consequences and the legal process of divorce–and especially the ways in which these two forces interact–are at the core of the ugly, protracted, and destructive divorce.

The bad divorce described above is steeped in ignorance. Conversely, the good divorce–and there is such a thing–is steeped in knowledge. It requires knowledge about the law and the legal system, the emotional process of divorce, and particularly the interaction between the legal and the emotional. It is only when divorcing people understand the divorce process from both perspectives (legal and emotional) that they can exercise real choice over their own behavior. If they can understand their long-term interests, they are better at curbing short-term impulses to act out their fears and anxieties. If they can separate myth from fact, they can better resist the siren song of those who urge them to fight. If they understand the legal system as it affects divorce, they are better equipped to hold their lawyers accountable and to resist the worst side effects of the adversarial system. And when divorcing people can act in the face of knowledge rather than ignorance and fear, they stand a much greater chance of achieving a good divorce that allows all family members to rebuild and thrive.

As a lawyer and mediator of many years' experience, I have devoted my career to helping people achieve good divorces. I have worked with more than 3,000 couples over the years and have acquired a broad perspective on how divorces evolve. And I have seen that the chances of a good divorce can be dramatically improved if the divorcing individual is educated appropriately early in the divorce. Much of what I do as a mediator is to educate my clients so they can gain control of their own behavior and thereby shape a constructive divorce. Toward that end, I wrote two books aimed at educating divorcing people about the emotional and legal processes of divorce.[1] Few weeks go by that I do

[1] *Getting divorced without ruining your life, second edition* (2001). New York: Simon & Schuster. *A man's guide to a civilized divorce* (2003). Emmaus, PA: Rodale Press.

not receive an e-mail thanking me for one of these books and telling me that it made a difference. This book is an extension of that mission, aimed not at divorcing individuals but at the therapists who are so well situated to help them.

I hope this book provides readers with the information and understanding to enable them to expand their practices and to prevent much of the mischief and gratuitous pain imposed on families by the adversarial system of divorce.

Acknowledgments

Few books come into being from the efforts of the author working alone. Several people provided critical assistance, and I want to thank them here. First and foremost, I want to thank Batya Yasgur, my friend and colleague, who provided invaluable assistance reorganizing the book at moments when I had gotten into a complete muddle. Without her painstaking work and critical analysis, the book would have likely been stillborn. I also want to extend special thanks to my editor, Jim Nageotte, of The Guilford Press, who endured my curmudgeonly muttering with humor and forbearance. It has been a distinct pleasure to work with him. Finally, a note of thanks is due to the thousands of clients who have shared their stories and lives while they worked their way through some of life's most challenging moments. The dignity, grace, and intelligence demonstrated by so many of them was the foundation of my conviction that good divorces are available to most divorcing couples.

Contents

Introduction

DIVORCE AND THE MISSION OF THE THERAPIST

Divorce has long been the subject of professional turf battles. Lawyers, accountants, financial planners, actuaries, mediators, and therapists all claim pieces of it. The lawyers, of course, claim most. Most divorce lawyers believe that other professionals should play only those roles explicitly delegated by the lawyer and under the lawyer's firm control. And when challenged, lawyers often make noise about "the unauthorized practice of law" and threaten sanctions against anyone with the temerity to claim an independent role. This can be intimidating to therapists who seek to provide couples with counseling surrounding divorce-related issues and who fear malpractice litigation.

From the therapist's viewpoint, such threats are unsettling, frustrating, and worrisome. Divorce is a major component of the practices of most therapists. With about two million people getting divorced each year, and other millions thinking about or recovering from divorce, there is a great deal of work for therapists helping clients cope with divorce.[1] Beyond the role they play in custody evaluations, which actually are required in only a small segment of divorce cases, therapists assist clients and families in dealing with the complex emotions that accompany every stage of divorce. I submit that therapists consistently fail to go far enough in their treatment of divorcing couples. But for their fear of treading into territory controlled by lawyers, therapists would help their clients in many ways that presently don't occur to them. There are dozens of points in a divorce at which decisions made

[1]Kreider, R. M. (2005, February). Number, timing, and duration of marriages and divorces: 2001. *Current Population Reports*, pp. 70–97.

in the "legal" sphere have enormous emotional consequences seldom anticipated by either clients or their lawyers. And there are also dozens of decision points at which clients make "emotional" choices that have tremendous legal consequences, also not anticipated by either the client or the professionals hired to help.

In this book I want to arm the therapist with the knowledge and understanding necessary to provide better guidance for clients. I want the therapist to have a better grasp of the law and legal procedures of divorce. I want to scrape away the mystique that surrounds the legal world and insulates lawyers from accountability as they make decisions that are emotionally destructive for divorcing people and their families. I also want the therapist to have a more systematic understanding of the way that the emotional process of divorce interacts with the legal process of divorce. Most of all, I want to embolden therapists to provide support and information to clients about all aspects of the divorce process–emotional, legal, and practical.

BACKGROUND

I have spent 25 years working with divorcing couples, first as a litigator, then as a litigator and mediator, and finally as a mediator exclusively. I have mediated at least 3,000 divorces. That means I have heard the stories of thousands of divorcing people, reviewed the financial problems of thousands of families, and worked with hundreds of lawyers, therapists, and other professionals. Much of what I discuss in this volume is based on the patterns of behavior I have observed repeatedly through the years. As a teacher of mediation, I have worked with and supervised hundreds of lawyers, therapists, and other professionals as they have endeavored to learn the craft of mediation. I have had a rich opportunity to learn about the cultures of each profession and how they interact with and view one another.

Over the years I have practiced, I have also observed historical changes in approaches to divorce–including the role that mediation can play in divorce proceedings. When I started practicing mediation, I was the only mediator in the state of New Jersey, dealing with a hostile bar and judiciary. I spent years collaborating with other lawyers and therapists as we organized state and national organizations and began the long and difficult task of changing the way people divorce in this country. The divorce mediation movement was perhaps the first time lawyers and therapists came together to launch a major professional reform. The two groups made uneasy partners, and a good deal of skirmishing between the two marked the early years of the movement. For many lawyers, any involvement by therapists in mediating divorces was initially denounced as the unauthorized practice of law. But over a period of 10 years, unauthorized practice became a dead issue in mediation. Almost every state now has numerous practitioners of mediation, of whom the majority are therapists rather than lawyers. At the beginning, there were only a few of us in the country. Now there are thousands of mediators practicing, and mediation has been adopted, at least in part, by many judicial systems. I was among the leadership in establishing the standards, ethics, and training for the field and worked with many hundreds of therapists of all persuasions along the way. It is my experience as practitioner, teacher, and frequent combatant that shapes the guidance and perspectives offered in this book.

THE INTERACTION OF LEGAL, EMOTIONAL, AND PRACTICAL PROCESSES

What makes divorce unique is that it involves a unique interaction of two processes: emotional and legal. There is an emotional process in which a couple begins with disillusionment, leading to a decision by at least one of them to end the marriage. Then there are the transitions of early separation and the construction of two households from the resources that formerly supported one. This generates acute anxiety for most divorcing people. For most people who are not wealthy, divorce requires economic retrenchment, which often generates acute conflict about who gets what and how much. All of this engenders fear of loss and acute feelings of anger, betrayal, humiliation, and loss of identity. Couples have to live through a legal process involving negotiation of a separation agreement and have to get used to new living arrangements. Over time, the intense feelings may begin to lessen as people get used to new routines. Finally, depending on how much dislocation was generated by the legal struggle, most divorced people settle down into their new lives within about 5 years of separation.

Divorce is also a legal process. We cannot obtain a divorce without the approval of the state in which we reside. The state requires that we resolve issues related to care of the children, the support of each spouse, and the division of marital property. Even when divorcing couples are in agreement about all these issues, it is difficult to get divorced without at least some involvement by lawyers. The procedural complexity of the legal system makes it impenetrable to all but the pluckiest of laypeople. And if the divorcing couple is not in agreement, then the role of the lawyers expands, and the involvement of two adversarial lawyers begins to have a greater impact on how the divorce evolves. In a contested divorce–one in which the parties disagree on essential issues–the litigation goes through stages leading from initial pleadings through pretrial motions, discovery, trial preparation, and, if the case does not settle, a trial in which a judge decides the issues and imposes the decisions on the couple. Almost all cases settle prior to trial, but the settlement invariably occurs on the eve of trial.

The manner in which the legal process is conducted and the manner in which it interacts with the emotional process shape the outcome of the divorce. Generally, the more intense the conflict, the more difficult it is for families of divorce to adapt well to the divorce. Intense conflict in divorce engenders intense bitterness that interferes with the ability of the parties involved to get on with their lives. We know from many sources[2] that the successful adaptation of children after a divorce is directly related to the level of conflict between their parents. People who divorce with a minimum of struggle and who emerge from the divorce feeling that the settlement is just and fair are usually able to wish each other well and move on without the emotional consequences of the hotly litigated divorce. Bitter divorces tend to go on indefinitely. In some states, it can take 4 years or more to complete the divorce. But even when completed, the bad divorce frequently spawns an endless process, as the couple returns to court year after year to fight over children and money.

Given that the legal and emotional processes of divorce interact, therapists must be prepared to be involved in the divorce from beginning to end, even at the risk of giving advice that stretches their traditional comfort zone. The compartmentalization of "emotional" issues to therapists and "legal" issues to lawyers has led to a fragmented and ultimately destructive experience for couples and families going through divorces. When a therapist avoids dealing with the processes of a client's divorce, he or she abdicates a legitimate therapeutic mission–guiding clients through the emotional ramifications and re-

[2]Heatherington, E. M., & Kelly, J. (2002). *For better or for worse: Divorce reconsidered.* New York: Norton.

percussion of a divorce–to lawyers, who are woefully ill equipped to make or guide decisions that shape the emotional lives of families. As we will see in Chapters 5 and 6, lawyers are trained to operate in an adversarial professional culture that undermines families and inhibits their capacity to heal emotionally. The legal training leads many lawyers unintentionally to fan the flames of hostility between divorcing partners. In the chapters to come, I will show how the legal culture evolved and how it clashes with the needs of families in contemporary divorce. I will demonstrate that the more contact divorcing couples have with the legal system, the worse off they will be, and the less reliant that couples are on the legal system, the better off they will be.

Finally, because divorce requires changes in living arrangements, it requires many practical decisions about housing, moving, employment, child raising, and careers, among other issues. All of these can have significant emotional ramifications. In the few cases that go to trial, a judge will decide most of these issues, but in the vast majority of cases, the divorcing couple must decide all these questions themselves. Because divorcing people have to make so many practical decisions that have emotional consequences, I contend that the therapist must be available to help guide practical decisions so that clients can decide wisely.

CHANGE AFFECTS THE ENTIRE FAMILY

The changes that are required by divorce inevitably affect each member of the family. Over the past 50 years, the concept of the "best interests of the child" has become part of the taken-for-granted reality of lawyers and the judicial system and is routinely invoked as a piety by lawyers trying to get a better deal for their clients. One purpose of this book is to reframe "the best interests of the child" to "the best interests of the family." It is important to understand that the "best interests of the child" makes sense only in an adversarial system in which the best interests of the child are defined as clashing with the best interests of the parent–or, in short, parent versus child. Salvador Minuchin, the grandfather of modern family therapy, once said that "divorce is not the death of a family. It is the reorganization of a family"[3] If we put the

[3]Minuchin, S. (1974). *Families and family therapy*. Cambridge, MA: Harvard University Press.

needs of all family members in a reasonable perspective, the decisions that emerge serve the best interests of the family. So, the priority attached to the needs of the children is the same as that attached to the needs of the parents. Sorting this out and helping clients maintain a balanced perspective that attends to the needs of all family members is a task for which most therapists are far more suited than most lawyers.

THE ROLE OF THE THERAPIST

Therapists can make a profound positive difference in the outcome of a divorce if they can overcome their timidity, stay with their clients throughout the process, and provide guidance not only about emotional and practical issues but also their relation to legal decisions. This may involve challenging some long-held notions of the role of therapists. Classically, the role of the therapist is not to "guide" so much as create a forum in which the client can make his or her own decisions. However, some concrete hands-on guidance is necessary when it comes to divorce. This includes providing information and, whenever possible, steering clients away from litigation unless it becomes a last resort and toward collaborative negotiation more likely to secure the welfare of the client's entire family.

I am aware that this expanded role may cause discomfort for some therapists. First, some may believe, however erroneously, that I am encouraging therapists to engage in the unauthorized practice of law and that they will get "sued" by the bar. In all my years of practice, and after contact with hundreds of therapists who have been actively engaged with divorcing couples throughout the country, I have never heard of a single therapist who has been sued for the unauthorized practice of law. I have also never heard of a single therapist who has ever been sued for malpractice by a client because the therapist gave bad advice about a divorce. To some degree, the fear that therapists have about lawyers and litigation is reflective of the general hysteria in the society about lawyers and "being sued." The perceived danger is vastly greater than the actual danger.

It is noteworthy that there are many other professions whose work requires providing clients with a significant amount of legal information. Architects, engineers, and accountants, for example, must interpret laws and legal codes for their clients. And it is an accepted principle of law that, when professionals advise clients about the law *incidental to their primarily professional role,* this does not constitute the unauthorized practice of law. In this book it is my objective to convince the reader that managing the emotional consequences of divorce is completely within the professional purview of therapists and that any incidental discussion of divorce law is fully permissible and well within the bounds of exemplary professional practice.

A second objection I anticipate from some therapists is that the kind of problem solving I advocate in divorce exceeds the traditional mission of therapists as healers and as facilitators of the clients' own decision making about their own lives. I submit that prevention of emotional harm is squarely within the role of healer. And I also submit that clients cannot make intelligent decisions when they are ignorant of the facts and burdened by misconceptions and myths about the issues. If helping clients and their families to survive the emotional hazards of divorce is not within the legitimate scope of a therapist's role, then I wonder just who should take responsibility for that task.

THERAPEUTIC CONTEXTS

To this point, I have spoken about "therapists" as if they were a homogeneous group. Of course, there are numerous therapeutic specialties and therefore numerous contexts in which a therapist is likely to intersect with divorcing couples.

School counselors may be asked to evaluate or counsel a child with academic or behavioral difficulties. It may emerge that the child's parents are going through a divorce and that the emotional turmoil at home is affecting the child's performance at school. Similarly, child and adolescent therapists may encounter divorcing parents through the emotional issues that the child brings into the therapy room. In both such cases, it is not only appropriate but critical for the therapist to meet with the parents and ascertain what is going on in the household surrounding the divorce. Once this information is obtained, it is equally important for the therapist to provide information and guidance to the parents so that they can make wise choices that support the successful functioning of the entire family, including the child who is the therapist's client. Most often, the therapist's primary role in this process will be to steer the couple away from litigation and refer them to a mediator instead.

Individual therapists are often privy to the client's dissatisfactions with a marriage, his or her plans to end the marriage, or the distress experienced if the spouse decides to end the marriage. Helping the client to make emotionally sound legal and practical choices is as critical as helping the client deal with the "pure emotions" that have so often been viewed as the essential core of therapy.

Marriage and family therapists might be the most important practitioners to have an impact on the course and outcome of a divorce. Many marriage counselors consider their role to be terminated when a couple announces the decision to divorce. They wish their clients well and tell them that it's time for them to consult lawyers. These therapists are exiting at arguably the most sensitive and crucial turning point–when the couple must start making numerous decisions that will have enormous repercussions on their mental health, the well-being of their children, their finances, and their living situation for many years to come.

There are other therapists who will find this book useful–for example, leaders of support groups for those going through divorce or children whose parents are divorcing, or pastoral counselors whose parishioners have sought marriage counseling. Whatever your particular therapeutic area of expertise and practice, this book will arm you with the information you need to be of maximum assistance to your clients. It is not the intention of the book to tell you how to conduct therapy. Nor, given the broad range of therapeutic modalities and strategies, would it be reasonable to suggest specific therapeutic scripts to deal with the problems raised in the book. I assume that each reader has his or her own way to execute the tasks suggested in helping clients through the divorce.

USING THIS BOOK

The purpose of this book is to provide therapists with the information they need to guide clients toward a good divorce. My experience has shown me that most divorcing couples are capable of ending their marriages constructively and peacefully, leading to a "good" divorce, and that many angry, bitter divorces ("bad" divorces) are avoidable. Steering clients toward a good divorce can be accomplished only if therapists understand the components of a good divorce and the interaction among emotional, legal, and practical processes. This book is organized accordingly.

Chapter 1 discusses the problem of mutuality–the difference between initiators and noninitiators and the impact of those differences on the divorce process. Chapter 2 lays out the components of good and bad divorces. Chapters 3 and 4 describe the emotional challenges that arise as couples decide to divorce and then separate. The next chapters deal with legal aspects of divorce and their impact within the emotional and practical realms. Chapters 5 and 6 discuss legal culture in general and divorce law in particular. Chapter 7 presents concrete guidance for helping clients to choose lawyers and mediators. Chapter 8 suggests ways to support clients through the negotiation process that is so central to the process of divorce. Chapters 9, 10, and 11 discuss the legal, emotional, and practical aspects of child support and alimony, custody and parenting, and the distribution of property. Chapter 12 is devoted to helping clients manage the economic problems usually associated with divorce. In Chapter 13 I discuss issues related to pulling together the final agreement and moving on to the formal divorce. Chapter 14 addresses how to help clients cope with problems that often arise after the divorce is over. I end with some concluding thoughts. The book contains many composite or actual case histories, with names and surrounding details disguised to protect the privacy of the individuals involved.

In totality, the book is designed to enable the therapist to assume an advisory role at virtually every stage of the divorce process.

1 Understanding the Problem of Mutuality

The first step in understanding the psychological dynamics of divorce is realizing that the decision to end a marriage is seldom mutual. Almost invariably one of the partners reaches the decision to divorce before the other, often after having thought about it for a very long time. The person who decides to end the marriage is called the initiator, while the other person is called the noninitiator. The initiator is the one who decides to divorce. This has nothing to do with who files in the court, as we will discuss later. The discrepancies between the initiator and the noninitiator create a dynamic that underlies virtually all the other aspects of the divorce. Understanding this issue of mutuality will better enable therapists to assist clients through the stages of the divorce process and the tasks that each member of the couple must undertake to achieve a good divorce.

This chapter is designed to introduce the issue of mutuality and explore how it plays out through the divorce process. We will also provide a basic overview of the stages and tasks involved in divorce. The subsequent chapters will provide more detailed guidance regarding therapeutic intervention at each juncture.

INITIATORS AND NONINITIATORS

Marriages erode rather than break. People who started off excited about each other and vowing eternal love do not simply have an epiphany one day and decide to end the relationship. Disillusionment sets in gradually, after many skirmishes have gone unresolved. People give up on marriages slowly, one disappointment at a time. After eventually reaching the conclusion that the marriage isn't going to improve, one or both parties may begin to fantasize an escape, and with enough practice the fantasy is transformed into a plan. Gradually, the initiator begins to accept the inevitability of the divorce.

In some cases, decisions are made but deferred until some event, usually involving the development of the children, has occurred. The divorce is put off until the youngest child enters school full-time or until a child graduates from high school. Then the initiator feels free to announce to the other that he or she wants a divorce. In a few cases, the announcement is made as a gesture to get the other spouse to change: the partner who is threatening the divorce really hopes that the other will meet his or her demands so that the marriage can continue. But in my experience with thousands of divorces, in most cases by the time the initiator says "I want a divorce," the marriage is genuinely dead. The feelings of attachment necessary to sustain a marriage have dissipated, and there is nothing left to support the relationship.

The partner who initiates the divorce has the clear psychological advantage. She (or he) has had time to come to terms with her disappointment over the failure of the marriage. She has had time to mourn and, more importantly, time to plan. As she reached the conclusion that the divorce was necessary, she was able to think through a scenario for ending the marriage. She has probably discussed her problem with others and likely confided her plans to some intimate friend. She has begun to plan for a new social life and perhaps a professional life. It is not uncommon for the initiator to start developing new friends separate from the spouse, to enroll in a graduate program to seek new credentials, or even to embark on an affair as reassurance that she is still attractive. Men may begin to spend more time at the office, expand their social circle, seek the companionship of women, and talk to their buddies who are divorced. All of these planning activities further the planning process for the divorce and advance the sense of detachment from the spouse.

It is the noninitiator who is at a clear psychological disadvantage in the beginning of the divorce. When the initiator breaks the news, the other spouse is somewhere on a continuum between resigned agreement and shock. If the two have been struggling for a long time and if they have had many discussions about their inability to repair the marriage, the announcement by a partner that he or she has decided to end the marriage may not be a surprise at all to the other. "Well, I was willing to try a while longer, but I can't argue with it. The marriage has been dead for a long time, and we probably ought to end it." Such a response makes the divorce decision mutual. As we shall see, the divorce has a greater chance of being amicable when it is mutual. More typically, however, the noninitiator is shocked and enraged. "I knew we were having troubles, but that doesn't mean we should be getting divorced. How can you go ahead and make such a unilateral and sudden decision about something so important?"

The noninitiator's disadvantage stems from the nature of change that comes with divorce. Take, for example, the typical middle-class family with two children. One or both of the parents will have to move to another home. All of the family members will have to retrench economically and spend less money. If the family has to move because the family home is no longer affordable, children may have to make new friends and possibly adjust to new schools. And the children may be unhappy about the divorce and have emotional struggles that require increased attention from parents–exactly at the time the parents are severely stressed and least able to give.

Each parent will have to reconstruct social and emotional lives. Many of the couple's friends may drop away. One or both of the parents may feel uncomfortable in the church they have attended and feel the need to find a new one. Each may have to negotiate dating, with all the awkwardness and discomfort that often entails. And if one or both of the parties finds a new mate and remarries, there are all the changes associated with creating new stepfamilies.

So, divorce involves significant challenges and often uncomfortable changes, all of which come at an emotional price. For the initiator who has had the time to think through the divorce, the painful changes and the losses associated with the divorce are offset by the advantages perceived as flowing from it. As one of my male clients expressed it, "When I moved out into my own apartment, I was worried that I would miss the kids so much–and I did. But the sense of peace I had and the sense that I was finally out from under all that misery and unhappiness made it worth it." Simply put, for the initiator, gains outweigh losses.

For the unprepared noninitiator, it will be just the opposite. For this person, there is nothing but losses. Whereas the initiator is optimistic, the noninitiator is pessimistic. The noninitiator is unprepared to look forward to the relief that will come from building something new, but simply experiences the divorce as stripping away all sense of security and even personal identity.

The noninitiator must have time to come to terms with the

divorce. Many bad divorces are caused by the demand that the noninitiator move faster than he or she is able to move. The early stages of divorce involve an acute sense of crisis. The noninitiator must be given time to grieve and recover from the sense of shock he (or she) feels. He needs time to take stock of what the divorce means to him, to recover from the feelings of abandonment, humiliation and, often, rage that are deeply felt early in the process. When the divorce moves ahead before both parties are ready, it may arouse a sense of panic in the noninitiator, who then seeks a lawyer to "protect" him. So, if an impatient initiator goes to a lawyer who encourages an early filing of a complaint for divorce, adversarial litigation is almost inevitable. As we will see later in the book, almost all divorces end with a negotiated settlement. Settlements cannot be negotiated until both partners are ready to negotiate and to plan their futures with a reasonably clear mind. It is impossible to negotiate when you are in a crisis state and unable to see anything but your own grief and fear. Compromises that would be unthinkable for the noninitiator early in the process will be possible once both partners are ready.

THERAPEUTIC GOALS

The mission of the therapist as a divorce begins is to monitor the manner in which it begins. The therapist may be treating the initiator, the noninitiator, or the couple when the initial decision to divorce is broached by the initiator. The tasks will be different depending on who is the client.

When the Initiator Is the Client

If the initiator has been in individual therapy, it is likely that the decision to divorce and the process leading up to that decision have likely been long-standing topics in therapy. The client has had ample opportunity to explore with the therapist the feelings that accompany the end of the marriage, work through the fears about the future, and explore scenarios for a future life. The task of the therapist in this situation is to help the initiator explore ways to conduct him- or herself to make it as easy as possible for the noninitiator to come to terms with the divorce. Although the initiator is the client, and obviously the therapist's main concern, the well-being of the noninitiating spouse has a profound impact on the well-being of the initiator/client. By increasing the chances of a healthy long-term outcome for the noninitiator and the children (if there are any), the therapist in the long run best serves his or her client. Thus, for example, the therapist may guide the client regarding what and what not to say. The client can be helped to form realistic expectations of the behavior of the other spouse and not to be provoked or overreact when the non-initiating spouse becomes upset and provocative. We will explore the details of breaking the news in Chapter 3. For now, I submit that management of this early stage by the initiator is critical and that appropriate early guidance from the therapist may make the difference between a good and a bad divorce.

When the Noninitiator Is the Client

When the noninitiator is the client, the task of the therapist is more complex. First, the therapist has to help the client work through the end of the marriage while coping with acute feelings of betrayal, rejection, and fear. The therapist counsels calm and encourages the client to take his or her time before reacting. In other words, the therapist advises the client to act counterintuitively and to show restraint. In some cases, the therapist already has a long-established relationship with the client and has been working with him or her on some of the very issues involved in the divorce. In other cases, the therapist sees the client for the first time when the client is referred for help with the crisis caused by the announcement of the other spouse. Of course, it is easier if the therapist has already established trust and rapport with the client, but the essential tasks remain the same—to facilitate the client's ability to gain perspective fairly quickly and to dissuade the client from premature legal action. The vulnerability of the client may motivate her (or him) to lunge at any offers of support and help, including those offered by lawyers who present themselves as rescuers and defenders, and family members and friends who encourage her to protect herself by engaging a lawyer as soon as possible. Enabling the client to feel less helpless and vulnerable involves educating her about the nature of divorce and helping her to develop realistic expectations about the needs of the other spouse. Noninitiators need to learn that time is a friend rather than a foe. Allowing time to adjust to the news and deal with the immediate emotional impact will not detract from strength but will contribute to it and enable the client to emerge empowered and clear-thinking.

When Both Partners Are Clients

In my experience, most middle-class couples try marriage counseling before accepting that their marriage must end. The therapist may have worked with the couple for some time before one partner decides on the divorce. Alternatively, the therapist may be consulted only after one partner has announced the divorce to the other. In the former case, the therapist knows the couple well and already has a developed rapport with them. In the latter case, the therapist must intervene in a crisis before rapport has been fully developed. In either case, the therapist has the opportunity to help the couple maintain control and to avoid the pitfalls of precipitous and destructive legal action. Although it may be necessary to speak to each member of the couple alone, when both partners are present, it can be easier to deal with the difference in readiness and mutuality and to help each understand the needs of the other.

Marriage counselors, like individual therapists, should advise the couple to take more time before making decisions about legal action. This may be met with surprise, especially if the couple has already been in therapy for a while. The initiator might feel that, by being in therapy, the noninitiating partner already has had plenty of time to adjust to the possibility of a divorce, and that the decision should come as no surprise. Impatient to move toward the new life that awaits, the initiator may feel tempted to hasten the legal process. But what few laypeople understand is that filing a suit for divorce invariably slows down rather than accelerates the divorce–often by a matter of years. On the other hand, the noninitiator may feel betrayed, concluding that the initiating partner has been attending counseling sessions only as a ruse and has been planning this all along. The shock and anger might motivate her to precipitously begin the legal process as a way of "getting back" at the partner. Both partners need to be reined in while they make their way through the stages and complete the emotional tasks that must be mastered at the beginning of divorce.

STAGES IN THE DIVORCE PROCESS

Divorce involves many practical decisions and psychological reactions that do not occur all at once. Instead, most divorcing couples go through a fairly predictable set of stages that unfold in time. While the couple as a unit goes through these stages, each party does so as well, and at his or her own pace. Understanding these stages enables a therapist to address the emotions that typically accompany each stage at the most appropriate juncture. Well-timed intervention can spell the difference between a rancorous divorce and an amicable one.

First Stage: The Decision to Divorce

The decision to divorce begins when one or both partners become disillusioned with the marriage and ends when both acknowledge that the marriage is over. I use the term "acknowledge" rather than "agree" because the noninitiator may be opposed to the divorce, even though he (or she) has accepted the fact that his partner has made an irrevocable decision. During this stage, initiators may feel overcome by guilt at inflicting pain, while noninitiators can feel victimized and filled with blame for the initiator. These emotions should be addressed in therapy. The time boundaries of this stage are discrete, because people respond at differing speeds. For example, an initiator might spend years mulling the decision to divorce before telling the spouse. But once the news is out, the process has begun.

Second Stage: Managing the Crisis

The second stage of divorce is one in which the couple begins to cope with the consequences of the decision to divorce. This is a difficult time, since emotions are intense and often volatile and the parties have not yet learned how to manage the inevitable conflicts. The issue of mutuality becomes even more critical at this stage. A reluctant noninitiator may respond to the initiator with punishing and threatening behavior. An impatient initiator may push the noninitiator too fast to make decisions about children, assets, and the marital home. The possibility for acting out by each spouse is very high, and as each begins to threaten or antagonize the other, distrust grows, and the parties can quickly retreat to lawyers and end up with an adversarial divorce.

The negative spiral can trigger acute anxiety and depression in both spouses, but particularly in the noninitiator. He may believe that his identity as a parent is threatened because he has heard all the horror stories about fathers losing their children. She may be worried that she will be socially ostracized because she has heard all the stories about middle-aged women who can't find husbands. He may mourn that he will lose half his savings or have to defer his retirement indefinitely because of the economic problems caused by the divorce. Or she may be frightened that she won't know how to take care of herself because she has never lived alone.

All of these problems and issues can be worked out over time. In fact, most people interviewed 5 years after a divorce report that they feel happier and more satisfied with life than they did when they were married. But in the early stages of the process, there has simply not been enough time for people to experience any potential benefits of breaking up. If they are able to get through this early period without intense struggles or challenges posed by the divorce, each will be able to get some perspective and approach the issues more creatively.

The sense of crisis typical of this stage can last from a month to a year, or even longer. It depends on how the spouses behave toward each other, because each is quite capable of prolonging the crisis experienced by the other. By the time this stage has ended, the shape of the divorce will be largely determined. For those couples who have managed well, each party will feel ready to get on with the separation and begin to solve the many practical problems associated with the transition. In contrast, for the couple that has engaged in an angry struggle, the divorce by this time is usually in litigation. A major goal of the therapist is to help the parties maintain reasonable, calm, and civil communication and to help them address the confusion, fears, and other emotions that surface during this stage.

Third Stage: Separation

Sooner or later a divorcing couple has to separate. It is my contention that the sooner separation occurs, the better off the entire family. When divorcing families continue to live together, everyone stays in limbo and things tend to get worse rather than better. I have observed that people cannot really relax or begin to heal until this separation occurs, but for a variety of reasons many couples find themselves living together for months and even years.

Unfortunately, the obstacles to separation are numerous. For most couples, the separation does not occur unless there is at least a tacit agreement on access to the children for the one moving out. There are also some formidable economic issues to resolve. The couple spends everything that they earn and perhaps more. There is not enough money in the budget to support a second residence unless they make significant changes in their present patterns of consumption. Most couples can find the money to effect a separation. In many cases it is the noninitiator who is resistant to spending the money, because, by arguing that there is no money, he or she can stave off an unwanted separation. The therapist has an important role here in helping the clients to weigh the damage to the mental health of the family caused by a continuation of living together versus the economic costs of a separation.

Separation is a critical time in the divorce, and communication can easily go awry. The therapist can make the difference here between a separation that develops smoothly and one that is filled with crisis and confrontation. We will explore this subject in detail in Chapter 4.

Fourth Stage: Negotiating the Agreement

As we will see in subsequent chapters, when an agreement has been negotiated after lengthy litigation, the lawyers generally do the negotiating, with the clients as passive onlookers to the process. These kinds of agreements tend to be grudgingly arrived at, with only limited commitment on the part of the spouses. About half of these agreements break down within 2 years, and then the parties are back in court fighting about children and support. In such a situation the therapist can, at best, help to limit the damage caused by this ongoing conflict. From a mental health perspective, the preferred method is for the agreement to be negotiated directly by the couple with the help of a mediator and the support of two advisory lawyers. Less desirable but still viable is negotiation with two lawyers who respect each other and are committed to resolving the issues peacefully without litigation. The therapist can help the couple approach the issue maturely by serving as translator and helping the client continually understand the concrete and future consequences of acting on immediate feelings. It is this process that promotes more rational and constructive behavior and collaborative negotiation.

The negotiation stage can last from a few months to a year or longer, depending on the behavior of the parties and their readiness to be finished. If they negotiate before both are ready, the process will take longer. Therapists can help clients to assess whether they are ready to resolve the issues. If either spouse is not ready, then some type of separation should be achieved with some temporary understanding about how children and money will be managed until both have reached a state of readiness. We will discuss this further in Chapter 4.

Fifth Stage: Rebuilding and Moving On

Once the separation agreement has been negotiated and signed by the spouses, each can focus on building a new life and helping the children to settle into new life patterns. Although the most difficult parts of the divorce are over, this stage is not without its dangers and pitfalls. Sometimes people suffer from "buyer's remorse," wondering whether they made a bad deal and made too many concessions. A spouse who sees the other living too well or seeming too happy may wonder why he or she is feeling so deprived. A husband who sees his wife dating other men may wonder if he was too generous in the settlement. New boyfriends and girlfriends can precipitate all sorts of anxieties. New parenting patterns can generate fear that the children are unhappy and cause sabotage of the other parent. Some of these issues can generate postdivorce conflicts, which we will cover at length in Chapter 14.

All of these conflicts are unsurprising and within the scope of "normal." But how they are handled will determine whether the family continues on the road to adjustment or is distracted by renewed battles. So, here too the role of the therapist as translator and a calming presence can be very useful to the clients.

STAGES ARE NOT DISCRETE

Although most couples pass through all the stages, the boundaries between each stage and the next are not starkly drawn. Both partners will not move at the same speed. Negotiations may begin in stage 2 or even in stage 1. One or both of the partners may begin to rebuild actively even before the settlement is negotiated. Clearly, negotiation of the settlement agreement is the central task for the couple. How well they perform this task will shape the future of the family. But divorce is seldom linear. A crisis of identity that seems resolved early on may surface later. Feelings of humiliation or anger may be suppressed for a while and then burst upon the scene. At each stage and between stages the partners have unlimited opportunity to step on each other's toes and begin an entire cycle of antagonism. So, the management of feelings and the education and coaching of the clients are continuous processes for the therapist.

THE EMOTIONAL TASKS OF DIVORCE

Divorce demands a set of tasks that the couple must confront and master. Divorce is a paradoxical experience in that divorcing people must master critical tasks both as individuals and as a couple. If one is to have a decent divorce, one must engage in collaboration with the very person one is divorcing. The couple must work together in order to live apart. There are parallel tasks, therefore, for each individual and for the couple as an entity. Both spouses must work their way through the individual emotional tasks in order for the couple to perform as well. And if either spouse fails in the individual emotional tasks, the couple is unlikely to succeed in mastering the joint tasks. The tasks facing a divorcing couple can roughly be categorized according to the stages we discussed above.

Stages 1 and 2: Tasks Involved in Managing the Decision to Divorce and the Crisis

- *Individual task:* Mourn the end of the marriage, accept the finality of the decision to divorce, and manage the feelings that flow from the decision. Here we are concerned with the ability of each spouse to let go of the fantasy that the marriage will continue. The initiator has usually completed this task by the time he or she announces the decision, but the noninitiator must go through the process, usually faster than did the initiator.
- *Couple's task:* Manage the issue of timing so that the initiator and noninitiator understand what each other needs, and respect those needs without demanding immediate resolution of all the issues.
- *Individual task:* Assume responsibility for one's own role in the demise of the marriage, a task that requires a certain degree of understanding of what happened. When an individual does this well, he or she is able to manage the feelings of pain, sadness, and loss. Managed poorly, these feelings manifest themselves as rage, panic, and a fruitless pursuit of vindication.
- *Couple's task:* Maintain civility and minimize angry exchanges in

which guilt, blame, and fault are assigned by each to the other. Manage an orderly separation as soon as possible.

- *Individual task:* Assist children with reassurance that things will be all right, and provide children with the additional comfort and support they need to manage the news of the divorce. This includes desisting from the temptation to recruit the children as allies or to influence their perception of the other parent.
- *Couple's task:* Develop a cooperative parenting arrangement in which both parents maintain robust relationships with the children and support each other's parenting.

Stages 3 and 4: Tasks Involved in Managing the Separation and Negotiation

- *Individual task:* Develop a viable plan for the future in a household separate from the spouse. This includes coming to grips with the tactical challenges of joint parenting, and accepting the necessary economic changes, changes in housing, and possible career development.
- *Couple's task:* Negotiate a separation agreement that maximizes the utilization of the family's resources and fairly distributes change to all family members, and that both spouses regard as equitable.

Stage 5: Tasks Involved in Rebuilding New Lives

- *Individual task:* Fully detach emotionally from the other spouse. Here the opposite of love is not hate but, rather, indifference. The individual no longer has strong feelings for the former spouse and wishes him or her well. This means that the individual is again emotionally available without the distractions of an unresolved marital relationship. The individual ceases to expect intimate dialogue with the spouse and ceases to turn to the spouse for emotional support or friendship.
- *Couple's task:* Adopt a civil and cooperative discourse around the children. The mode of communication resembles the communication style one would use with a colleague: one of respect, cordiality, and an absence of intimacy.
- *Individual task:* Build a new social life either as a successful single person or with a new intimate partner. Here the individual finds a successful new social equilibrium that leaves him or her feeling a modicum of emotional satisfaction with life.

• *Couple's task:* To provide continuing support to the other as a parent and to support the children as they adapt to the new relationships of each parent. This includes a continuation of collaborative problem solving when life changes require the negotiation of changes in the arrangements of the parties. The parties have now ceased to be a couple but have only a businesslike and cooperative relationship for raising children.

THE ROLE OF THE THERAPIST

The role of the therapist is to guide clients through these stages and tasks so that they can achieve a good divorce. Therapists not only can continually help clients identify what they feel at each stage but can also assist the client in predicting the consequences of acting on those feelings. The therapist can also help the client find reasonable interpretations of the behavior of the other spouse to minimize attribution of malice when the spouse's behavior is troubling. Generally, the therapist who is familiar with divorce can help normalize feelings and behavior and help the client keep his or her eye on long-term interests. Finally, the therapist can help the client explore the emotional consequences of legal strategies and tactics so that the client is not led blindly into destructive litigation. I find that a common refrain of those who are going through bad divorces is that "my life just feels that it is totally out of control." With the help of an educated therapist, clients should be able to maintain more control and therefore have richer choices.

2 What Is a Good Divorce?

A "good divorce" may sound like an oxymoron, but it is not unrealistic. To accomplish this goal, both parties must engage in emotional, legal, and practical behaviors that are difficult, even counterintuitive, at times. These behaviors can be learned and acquired with the help of a skilled therapist who is familiar with the psychological and legal dynamics of divorce and willing to guide couples through the process.

One way of understanding the therapist's role is to recognize that there are two aspects to the emotions that beset individuals going through divorce. The first is a response to the *fact* of divorce. The failure of a relationship causes hurt feelings, anger, fear of loss, and a host of other emotions that accompany change and dislocation. But it is important to distinguish between the feelings that arise from the *fact* of the marital failure and the feelings that arise from the *way* the divorce is transacted. When a divorce is characterized by acrimony, recrimination, and distrust, a second layer of pain and fear is added to the first, and a bad divorce is likely to ensue.

By the time a couple has decided to divorce, there is probably little that you as a therapist can do to alter the fact that the marriage has failed and a divorce is forthcoming. It is your role to provide support, help clients understand what has happened, and provide reassurance that the client will come through intact. These do not change the fact—they merely enable your client to cope with it effectively. But you can have a profound impact and actually change the way your clients get divorced by presenting to them the concept of a good divorce and providing them with the guidance and tools to accomplish this end. You can offer calm analysis of choices and encourage them to stay in con-

[1]See also the widely read book *The Good Divorce: Keeping Your Family Together When Your Marriage Falls Apart* by Constance Ahrons (New York: HarperCollins, 1994; revised and updated 1998) and my previous book *Getting Divorced without Ruining Your Life* (New York: Simon & Schuster, 1992; revised and updated 2001).

trol instead of surrendering to a destructive adversarial system. An effective therapist must have a focused vision of what constitutes a good divorce in order to help clients to achieve this outcome.

A good divorce consists of six components, which are listed in Sidebar 2.1. We will elaborate on them in greater detail later in this chapter, but first we will bring the seemingly remote idea of a good divorce to life by presenting you with two contrasting case histories and the role of the therapist in each scenario.

CASE STUDY: DICK AND TAMMY

Dick and Tammy are divorcing after 15 years of marriage. Dick is employed as a lending officer by a large bank and earns $90,000 a year. Tammy had been a registered nurse but quit 11 years ago when Chip, their first child, was born. A second child, Mandy, arrived 4 years later, and Tammy settled into the role of traditional homemaker.

Several years ago, Tammy began to feel that she and Dick were growing apart. Dick's long hours at the office left her alone with the children much of the time, and she felt abandoned. Even when he was around, she felt that he didn't take sufficient interest in her and was not emotionally expressive. At her request, the couple entered marriage counseling with Dr. Jones, who had been recommended by Tammy's best friend. But after

---

Sidebar 2.1. Elements of a Good Divorce

1. The couple is no longer tied to each other by bonds of mutual love or mutual hatred. They are emotionally divorced.
2. Both members of the couple have rebuilt their lives, and their new circumstances are fulfilling and satisfying.
3. Both think the divorce agreement is fair and that they need not devote further energy to seeking vindication.
4. They retain the ability to cooperate as parents and continue to function as a team, with good communication and effective systems of problem solving around the needs of the children.
5. The children are comfortable in both households. Neither parent undermines the other parent's household, and both parents give children permission to feel at home in either household.
6. The former spouses can resolve disputes themselves or through mediation as circumstances change within the family.

---

3 years of counseling, Tammy continues to feel that Dick will never meet her emotional needs and decides to divorce. Dick is resistant to a divorce because he thinks Tammy's dissatisfaction does not constitute sufficient reason to put the family through the trauma it will entail. But Tammy convinces him that her decision is irrevocable, and he reluctantly resigns himself to the divorce. The counselor expresses his regret at the decision, wishes the couple well, and terminates therapy.

COMMENTARY: This is a typical scenario of a divorce. Unfortunately, what is also typical is that the counselor, whose original mission had been to help the couple repair their marriage, bows out at this critical time–when a bolder view of his role could have saved the couple from the bad divorce that follows.

First Major Decision: Should Dick Leave?

Dick has accepted that Tammy will be the parent of primary residence. That is, she will continue to be the daily administrator of the lives of the children. He knows that he and she will eventually be living in separate dwellings but feels it unfair for Tammy to tell him to leave. "She wants the divorce; let her be the one to go." Tammy insists that it doesn't make sense for her to leave because she is the primary caregiver, and if she moves out, the children will have to go with her–meaning that the second residence will have to be larger than they can afford. "Why uproot the kids?" asks Tammy. "It's just common sense that you should be the one who moves."

Dick consults a divorced friend at work, who tells him he had the same situation, and that his lawyer had told him not to leave–that if he left he would be giving up a valuable bargaining chip in the divorce struggle that was sure to ensue. His friend's lawyer had said that staying in the house would put pressure on his wife to make concessions and get the whole case settled as a condition of his going. The friend gives Dick his lawyer's name and number, and Dick calls the lawyer.

What the friend does not tell Dick is that he had had a long and contentious divorce, that he and his ex-wife cannot even look at each other now without getting angry, and that they are still embroiled in constant conflict.

When Dick consults the lawyer, he receives the same advice as his friend. "Don't move. If you move out before the divorce is finalized you just encourage your wife to drag her feet and to take a harder line."

Feeling he has no alternative, Dick informs Tammy that he is staying in the house until their divorce is finalized. He suggests that if she wants him to move out, she'd better make as many concessions as possible to expedite the process.

COMMENTARY: Dick's decision to stay in the house signals to Tammy that she is in for a hard struggle and that Dick has come under the sway of his lawyer. To Tammy this means that she had better hire a tough lawyer to deal with Dick's lawyer, lest she get "screwed." In other words, Tammy interprets Dick's behavior as a declaration of war. It also means that the atmosphere in the house will become increasingly rancorous, with the two spouses locked in a spiral of ever increasing distrust and hostility. The children will be forced to live with two angry, depressed parents who are unable to give them the reassurance and emotional support that they need.

Dick is not a bad person. He just has a shortage of good advice. If he had an opportunity to think through the emotional consequences of his decision or to talk to a fair-minded and knowledgeable therapist, he might well decide to move out as an investment in the mental health of the family. So far, the only advice he has had is from his lawyer.

Ironically, the lawyer has not given him any "legal" advice. There are no legal consequences of Dick's move. Contrary to popular myth, Dick does not forfeit any property rights by moving, as we will see in Chapter 4. What the lawyer has given Dick is strategic advice related to the lawyer's assumption about how the settlement negotiation will evolve. Whether the lawyer has any explicit training in negotiation strategy is dubious. That the lawyer has no training in family psychology is a near certainty. So, unless Dick receives good advice from a therapist, he has no way of knowing that the emotional costs of his decision far outweigh any hypothetical negotiating advantage. Unfortunately the counselor, who could have offered educated guidance about the impact of Dick's decision on the family's mental health, has refrained from remaining involved because his perceived role has ended.

Second Major Decision: Should Tammy Go Back to Work?

Dick and Tammy have a financial problem. For years the couple has been spending more than Dick earns. They would run up credit card debt and then take a home equity loan to consolidate the debt. They have been increasing their mortgage balance every 2 years but are approaching their borrowing limits. Moreover, their equity in their house has decreased, and each is worried that he or she will have insufficient capital to start over. When Dick tells Tammy that she has to cut back on spending or get a job, she becomes angry and counters that it is his responsibility to "support her in the manner to which she has become accustomed." Dick now threatens to cut back on support unilaterally.

When Tammy discusses the problem with a friend, she learns that a local doctor is looking for an office nurse and that she could probably get the job even though she has been out of nursing for 11 years. Out of curiosity she calls the doctor's office and is invited in for an interview. She is surprised and happy to be offered a job. That evening, she shares the good news with her sister, who advises her against taking the job. "You'll endanger your chances to get alimony from Dick," the sister says ominously. "You'd better talk to a lawyer before doing anything rash."

Tammy's lawyer confirms her sister's fear. "When we go to trial," says the lawyer, "you may get less alimony if you are employed. We have a good chance of convincing the judge that you need to stay home with the children, and then Dick will have to pay you a substantial amount of alimony."

Tammy had been seeing a therapist, Dr. Toby, for many years, including the years in which she and Dick were in counseling together. She leans on Dr. Toby for emotional support. Now, Tammy consults the therapist about her dilemma of whether or not to take the job. Dr. Toby says that this is a legal issue, and is reluctant to give Tammy advice on this subject. "It is beyond my purview," the therapist says.

Tammy turns down the job. Each month the financial deficit becomes larger until finally Dick refuses to pay the mortgage. This precipitates a crisis, and the couple retreat to their lawyers for rescue.

COMMENTARY: Once again, we see a decision based on a litigation strategy with no understanding or consideration of the emotional consequences. For this couple, like most middle-class couples, available income is less than projected expenses. There is no question that the couple must reduce spending, increase income, or burn through all their savings and face eventual bankruptcy. How Tammy decides to handle the problem will determine how Dick interprets her intentions. If he sees that she is trying to help and to cooperate, he will be inclined to cooperate in return. If he believes she is simply trying to get all she can get without regard to fairness, then he will not cooperate any further than he is compelled to by a judge.

It is interesting to note that Tammy is initially inclined to take the job. It is regrettable that she decides not to do so at this time because eventually she will have to go back to work, as there is no other way for her to afford the lifestyle she seeks. Moreover, the job would have been good for her self-esteem and her sense of independence. The reinforcement she would have received from using her skills and knowledge and from contact with other professionals would have enhanced a sense of professional identity.

A competent therapist would make this clear in a way that would make sense to Tammy as a person. The therapist would help her weigh the impact of the lawyer's advice to stay home against the advantages of taking the job. But in this instance her therapist abdicates her responsibilities, claiming that this is a legal rather than an emotional process and therefore falls outside her domain. So, Tammy relinquishes a good opportunity. She trusts her lawyer, because she has no other information and the lawyer appears to be an expert. Sadly, her trust is misplaced. The lawyer has not told her that there is a very high probability that the case will settle before trial and that refraining from taking employment will play no role in a judge's decision because a judge will never get to decide the case. This strategy has poisoned the atmosphere and impeded the ease of reaching a settlement.

A Toxic Atmosphere and Its Repercussions

Dick and Tammy are both stuck. Dick refuses to leave, and Tammy has refused to get a job to relieve the financial burdens. The atmosphere in the house becomes ever more rancorous as each seethes about the intransigence of the other. Communication becomes curt and cold, and the parties rarely talk. Tammy asks Dick to at least move out of the bedroom, and he responds that if she wants to move out she can, but he is not budging. After weeks of sleeping in the same bed with an angry spouse, Tammy can't take it any more and starts sleeping in the den. She also stops doing Dick's laundry or preparing dinner for him. Family meals cease to exist, and when Dick comes home from work the kitchen is an unpleasant place as the two bump into each other while preparing dinner.

The children feel the tension. Mandy starts to have trouble concentrating in school, and Tammy gets a call from the school's guidance counselor, who has been contacted by Mandy's teacher. "Mandy tells me there's a lot of tension at home," the counselor says, advising Tammy to "reduce the stress" so as to enhance Mandy's school performance. Tammy blames Dick for prolonging the stress and demands that he move out so the family can calm down. He angrily refuses.

One night after a particularly ugly fight, Dick storms out of the house. In anger, Tammy double-bolts all the doors so that Dick will not be able to get back in. When Dick returns home at 1:00 A.M., he is enraged to find himself locked out. He tries to call Tammy from his cell phone, but she refuses to pick up. In frustration, Dick finally breaks a window to get into the house. As soon as he does, Tammy calls the police, who come promptly. Because the state in which Dick and Tammy live has strict domestic violence laws, the police remove Dick from the house, and Tammy is advised to file a domestic violence complaint. She complies, and Dick is told to stay out of the house until a judge can conduct a hearing.

The next day, Tammy goes to her lawyer and tells him that she wants to keep Dick out of the house. The lawyer advises her to file for divorce immediately so the court can exercise jurisdiction. He suggests that she file on fault grounds—meaning, she must make allegations that Dick has harmed her in some way. Filing on fault grounds expedites the process of a divorce because the only nonfault grounds for divorce are that the couple are living separately, and obviously Dick and Tammy have not separated. The lawyer asks her for a list of all the mean and nasty things Dick has done over the years so that he can cite them in the complaint for divorce.

Although Tammy is reluctant to say negative things about Dick, she decides that she needs to listen to her lawyer, and so she writes 10 paragraphs in which she describes every time Dick has said something hurtful to her and every time he has been insensitive. Her lawyer drafts a complaint for divorce and files it with the court. A few days later the sheriff serves Dick with the complaint at his office. Having the sheriff show up in front of all his coworkers is very embarrassing to Dick, and when he reads the complaint he feels humiliated that Tammy has said such negative things about him in a public document.

Dick consults his lawyer that afternoon. The lawyer reads the complaint and expresses outrage. He tells Dick he needs to strike back as hard as he can so that Tammy will not start to think she is in a position of power. He advises Dick to counterclaim and to file a complaint alleging all the acts of cruelty that Tammy has committed. He also advises Dick to empty all the joint accounts. "Better get your hands on that money before she does," he says grimly.

So, that afternoon Dick follows his lawyer's advice. First he drafts his own version of a complaint for extreme cruelty in which he characterizes Tammy as a sloppy housekeeper who is lazy and chronically unpleasant. According to his complaint, she has been emotionally cold and has denied him sex for years, has been unsupportive of him in his career, and has alienated friends and relatives. The paragraphs he delivers to his lawyer are promptly incorporated in an answer and countercomplaint, which are duly filed and delivered to Tammy's lawyer.

The next day, Tammy is shocked when she goes to the bank to withdraw money, only to discover that Dick has emptied their joint account. In a panic, she calls their stockbroker and discovers that Dick has also moved the funds in that account into an account in his name only. She immediately calls for an appointment with her lawyer and is further chagrined when she arrives at his office and sees a copy of Dick's countercomplaint that her lawyer had received that morning. "How could Dick say such things about me?" she cries. "This is so humiliating."

The next day Tammy's lawyer files a motion in the court asking for emergency relief because his client has no money. He asks the court to hear this motion for temporary support, to freeze the marital assets, and to find that, because Dick had committed an act of domestic violence, he be permanently excluded from the home.

Two days later they all appear in court. After hearing the testimony, the judge rules that all the marital funds be frozen and that the parties be allowed access to funds only when they agree through their lawyers to a distribution. The judge also orders Dick to pay all the expenses and to pay Tammy an additional $300 a week as support. Tammy is pleased with that part of the judge's ruling. But she is displeased when the judge finds that Dick had not committed an act of violence against Tammy and refuses to order him out of the house.

COMMENTARY: Dick and Tammy have been living in an intolerably tense situation. The legal fight that follows an exaggerated domestic violence complaint is completely predictable. The situation is compounded by Tammy's lawyer, who advises her to immediately file for divorce rather than seek a negotiated resolution, although he knows that the eventual outcome will be a negotiated settlement–but only after Tammy and Dick have spent thousands of dollars, endured years of limbo, and have been wholly alienated from each other. This destructive process begins with the premature filing of a complaint before a settlement is negotiated.

The preferred way to proceed in a divorce is to file documents with the court only after a settlement has been negotiated. A divorce filed after a settlement has been negotiated goes onto the court's uncontested list–meaning that the court acknowledges there is no fight and the divorce proceeds smoothly. By contrast, when the complaint is filed before a settlement is negotiated, the divorce goes onto the contested list, alerting the court that it must step in to supervise a struggle. The court then begins the litigation process, and the financial and interpersonal costs start to accrue rapidly. Although there are some divorces in which an early filing is necessitated by genuinely abusive behavior on the part of one of the spouses, most divorces can be resolved by negotiation before any filing with the court takes place.

Another typical and destructive piece of advice comes from Dick's lawyer, who suggests that he retaliate against Tammy by withdrawing money from their joint accounts. This tactic backfires against him and adds to the vicious cycle that is developing.

Dick and Tammy's divorce is now only 1 week old, but already they are in serious trouble. Here is a summary of their present state:

- They have spent $12,000 on legal fees and wiped out almost half of their savings.
- Each has been enraged and humiliated by the other, and any semblance of trust and goodwill between them has been destroyed.
- Each has learned to talk only through lawyers and has been rendered completely dependent on the legal system for the resolution of any conflict.
- They are locked in the house together for the indefinite future, and they despair of ever regaining control over their lives. Neither can foresee anything but years of litigation and the liquidation of all their savings.

- Neither can begin to heal from the end of the marriage and rebuild their lives.
- Their children are forced to live in this hothouse of anger for the indefinite future. Mandy's school performance has already been adversely affected, and undoubtedly the toll on the children's emotional and academic well-being will continue to mount.

The Settlement and the Divorce

It is 2 years before the case is scheduled for trial. During that time, Dick and Tammy remain frozen in an intolerable set of conditions. The family endures 2 years of limbo, in which everyone becomes more despondent and depressed. Neither Tammy nor Dick can date or begin a new life. They talk only through their lawyers, but it costs several hundred dollars in legal fees every time. So, as a practical matter, all communication ceases. Tammy loses 2 more years from her career and Dick lives a lonely, isolated life. The children's mental health deteriorates. Mandy fails several courses, and Chip develops significant behavioral problems. Each lawyer combs through the personal and financial details of the other's client in a discovery process that never seems to end.

Finally, the case is scheduled for trial, and the judge requires a settlement conference. The conference goes on all morning, with the clients sitting in the hall and the lawyers shuttling in and out of the judge's office. At the end of the morning the lawyers meet with their respective clients. "We have reached a settlement. This is what the judge suggests, and in my experience it's not a good idea to go to trial once this judge has made his settlement suggestions. I recommend that you accept the settlement even though we aren't getting everything we want." And so, in an anticlimactic ending, the case is settled.

COMMENTARY: The terms of the settlement are similar to the terms that would have been reached 2 years earlier—except that Dick and Tammy have wasted $80,000 that they could not afford, and are emotionally and financially exhausted. Their prognosis for the future is poor because they have no means to communicate about issues involving their children, and both feel so burned that their fears and suspicions will be carried over into their next relationships. Their children have been subjected to turmoil and have suffered as a result.

Epilogue

Five years later, Dick and Tammy remain embroiled in litigation that never seems to end. Mandy's poor school performance has necessitated hiring expensive tutors and child psychologists, and the couple has been fighting over who is responsible for paying the bills. Dick believes Tammy is "pampering" Mandy and that she needs to "snap out of it" without the involvement of mental health professionals. He continues to blame Tammy, because it was she who wanted the divorce. Chip's behavior has deteriorated, and he has dropped out of school. His disrespect and contempt for rules make both parents dread his presence.

Tammy dates several men, but all of them are deterred by Chip's surliness and by Mandy's neediness, so Tammy goes through a series of dismal rejections. Dick remarries, but his new wife does not like the children, nor do they like her. Tammy goads them in their dislike and criticizes Dick's parenting. The stresses posed by ongoing litigation and by demanding children strain Dick's new relationship, and his wife starts talking about moving out.

COMMENTARY: Neither Dick nor Tammy is settled in their new lives, as they continually return to court to fight new battles and remain linked by mutual hatred. Their children become destructive forces in the context of rebuilding their new lives. They have had a bad divorce.

THE THERAPIST'S ROLE IN A GOOD DIVORCE

A favorite therapist of mine used to ask, "For what problems is this divorce a solution?" Clearly, Dick and Tammy have been unable to address any of the problems for which their divorce was supposed to be a solution. Moreover, they have created numerous additional problems for themselves and for the children that they are now in no position to solve. They are much worse off than when they began. And theirs is not a particularly unusual case. Neither of them is a bad person, and neither ever wanted to injure the other. They have followed the advice of lawyers who themselves are unable to anticipate the emotional consequences of their legal strategies and who see nothing wrong with the scenario that they have wrought.

Tammy and Dick's difficulties were caused by their inability to manage the initial transitions required by divorce. There were two critical problems they needed to address: how to separate amicably and quickly, and how to manage the financial strain that inevitably comes with middle-class divorce. But they did not address them, and acted on flawed advice from their attorneys.

What if they had remained in marriage counseling with Dr. Jones even after they decided to divorce, and Dr. Jones had understood the process of divorce? How might that have affected the outcome?

Dr. Jones would have moved to educate both spouses about the nature of divorce and would have normalized the feelings each client was having. He would have addressed Dick's anger and sense of rejection, which are typical reactions of the noninitiator. He would have advised Tammy to allow Dick to come to terms with the new circumstances without pressuring him. Dick's reluctance to leave the house would have been discussed in terms of what was best emotionally for each spouse and for the children. The financial obstacles to such a move would have been explored, and the couple would have been encouraged to be creative in finding ways to finance the move. Tammy's ability to go back to work, at least part-time, would have been explored, and Tammy would have had an opportunity to consider employment without pressure from Dick or misguided concerns about how her employment would affect her settlement. And, finally, the therapist would have discussed the alternatives for managing the divorce with the couple. He would have recommended mediation. If the couple felt mediation was not for them, Dr. Jones would have discussed the importance of choosing lawyers who were psychologically sophisticated and were both committed to nondestructive divorce.

This guidance would have made a critical difference for Dick and Tammy and would have helped them get through the beginning stages of the divorce without the destructive spiral that ensued. It would require that the therapist have the vision and leadership capacity to reassure each spouse that together they could manage the divorce decently without relinquishing their concerns and self-interest. They would have been provided an understanding of how each decision made at the outset of divorce would either open or close opportunities to solve problems in the future and achieve goals for a new life. All of this would have been within the proper scope of a marriage counselor's legitimate role.

Tammy's individual therapist, consulted later, also missed an opportunity. Had she been more knowledgeable about divorce and less fearful of overstepping her limits, she would have helped Tammy realize that taking a job would be good not only for family finances but also for her own personal growth. She might have helped steer Tammy in less destructive directions at several stages of the process and would have recommended mediation. The school guidance counselor likewise failed to offer useful interventions. She vaguely talked about the importance of "reducing stress" in the household but never suggested concrete measures to accomplish this aim.

Let's contrast the case of Dick and Tammy with the case of Bill and Karen.

CASE STUDY: BILL AND KAREN

Bill and Karen have been married for 20 years. Bill is 47, and Karen is 45. They have three teenage children. Bill is a systems analyst for a defense contractor and earns $110,000 a year. Karen is a teacher by training but stopped teaching when their youngest child was born, because the needs and requirements of child rearing were too great for her to manage along with a job. They have gotten by on Bill's salary but have not managed to save much.

For several years Karen has felt restless and uneasy in the marriage. She has begun to see a therapist. As she has explored her discomforts, she has become increasingly aware that the marriage had been subordinated early on to the needs of the children and never recovered from this shift in priorities. Although Karen and Bill rarely fight, they do not seem to have much in common anymore either. Lovemaking has diminished over the years, and sex, when it occurs at all, has become perfunctory and unsatisfying.

Now that the children have become more independent, Karen has started thinking of reestablishing a career. Three teenagers still require supervision but do not require the same amount of daily care as younger children. So, Karen signs up for some courses at a local college. She has long thought about becoming a lawyer and wants to take a few courses in law and government to see if she likes it.

Not only does she like her classes, but she also enjoys the company of other students and looks forward to going out for coffee after class with them. During her second semester, she meets a man who is auditing a course on constitutional law and starts to look forward to having coffee with him after class. Karen feels a little guilty about her friendship with Craig and never mentions it to Bill.

About this time, Karen's dissatisfaction with her marriage intensifies. She finds herself being temperamental and impatient with Bill, who tolerates Karen's behavior only because he thinks it is some "woman's thing" that will pass in time. But as Karen becomes ever more distant, Bill finally confronts her and is surprised to learn that Karen is unhappy with him. Although he had never felt enthusiastic about counseling and has not understood why Karen sees a therapist, he suggests that the two of them find a marriage counselor and try to fix whatever is wrong. Karen agrees, although she does not have much optimism about the enterprise.

Bill and Karen start therapy with Dr. Levy and continue their sessions for a few months. Each keeps repeating what he or she wants from the other. Karen says she wants more attention and romance and wants Bill to court her more. She wants Bill to be an intimate partner, not just a roommate. Bill says he just wants peace. He wants Karen to settle down and stop complaining. He says he will try to be more "emotional," although he is not sure what that means. Counseling does not accomplish much, since neither is truly committed to the process. Finally, Dr. Levy begins to ask some difficult questions. Do they really want to be married, and are they willing to do the hard work to make a success of the therapy? In response, Karen blurts out that she really wants a divorce. She does not think she can be happy with Bill and wants to be free to pursue a new life.

Bill is taken by surprise by Karen's revelation, and after a little thought starts to feel ambushed. He believes that Karen had never really intended to work on the marriage but was just using the therapy to find a safe place to break the news that she wants a divorce.

At this point the therapist intervenes. She suggests that the couple spend at least one or two sessions talking about the decision to divorce. She says that if they do proceed toward a divorce she would remain available to help them manage the emotional aspects of the divorce. She also says that, in her experience, couples can stay in control of the divorce if they each commit to a cooperative process. She invites them to call her in the days ahead and wishes them well.

COMMENTARY: At this point, much as Dr. Levy would like to help the couple to have a successful marriage, months of counseling have made it clear that the marital relationship has failed and that the couple will divorce. The therapist accepts this and offers to help Bill and Karen deal with the fact *that there will be a divorce. But–*

equally important–she offers to provide concrete guidance about the way *that the divorce will take place.*

Bill leaves the session very angry with Karen and refuses to talk to her for days. But after a week, he tells Karen that he will not try to hold her in a marriage that she does not want and suggests that she move out. He says that he can manage the children and that since she is the one who wants the divorce, she should move out and get a job. Karen is furious. "I've devoted my entire adult life to these kids and to making a home for them, and I'll be damned if I'm going to just move out and leave all my hard work behind!"

COMMENTARY: At this point, Bill and Karen are experiencing very similar emotions to those of Dick and Tammy. Bill feels betrayed by Karen and does not understand what he has done wrong. He regards her as fickle and untrustworthy, because she is prepared to violate her marriage vows in the name of some nebulous idea of happiness. Karen feels that Bill is emotionally stunted in his ability to express affection and that he will never change. She regards his anger as an ominous sign of how he might become nasty. They are both angry and distrustful of each other.

The Atmosphere Becomes Tense; Lawyers Are Consulted

Both Bill and Karen seek solace and support from friends. Each receives the typical advice: "Don't make any concessions. Be prepared to fight. Get the toughest lawyer you can find." Karen consults a lawyer suggested by a friend. The lawyer tells her that she will get permanent alimony and custody of the kids if she "just waits it out." She is also told that she will be able to stay in the house until the youngest child graduates from high school. But the lawyer advises her to expect at least a year in the house with Bill because there is no way to force Bill out until a judge gives her exclusive possession when they go to trial–which would be in about a year. Karen is upset because she can't imagine the family living so long in the tense environment that is developing. She is sure that this type of atmosphere must be emotionally destructive to everyone, especially the children, and she wonders if her lawyer's advice is really sound.

Bill also seeks legal advice. His lawyer tells him not to move out.

He adds that it is reasonable to expect Karen to resume teaching in order to help support herself and the kids. When Bill tells the lawyer about rumors he's heard that Karen has been seeing some guy at the college, the lawyer suggests hiring a private detective to follow Karen and gather proof of her infidelity, which would give him leverage in settlement discussions. The lawyer says that under the circumstances and considering the ages of the children, Bill has a good chance of winning a custody fight and getting both the kids and the house.

Bill is troubled by the lawyer's attitude. He recognizes that following the lawyer's advice might get him some advantage–but at what price? Sure, he's angry and would like some sense of vindication, but what would it do to the kids to have to live through such a battle? And where would the money come from to pay legal fees? They don't have much savings, and the only way to come up with the $20,000 the lawyer estimates it would cost to go to trial would be either to liquidate part of his retirement fund or to take out some of the equity from the house. Bill guesses that Karen is facing the same financial dilemma. Could they really waste this much money and still be able to finance the kids' college education?

COMMENTARY: Both Bill and Karen are having misgivings about the scenario that their respective lawyers are presenting, and each is uneasy about the enormous financial commitment that is being asked of them. They are showing maturity and good judgment when they hesitate and do not sign the retainers but decide to think it over first.

The Marriage Counselor Helps Bill to Manage His Emotions

Bill feels at a loss. All his family and friends have goaded him on in his efforts to find an aggressive lawyer who will be a "real fighter," but he continues to wonder if his long-term interests will really be served by taking the lawyer's advice. Then he remembers that the marriage counselor had offered to help. Wondering whether and how a marriage counselor can be useful in a divorce, he calls her.

Dr. Levy agrees to see him. She also suggests that he inform Karen of his appointment with her and that he invite Karen to join the session. Bill takes Dr. Levy's advice, and it seems as though Karen actually welcomes the news. However, she declines to have a joint session with Bill and Dr. Levy, saying that she will work with her own therapist and see Dr. Levy later if the need arises.

Bill goes to see Dr. Levy. After listening to his account, she explains that the key difference between Bill's and Karen's reactions to the upcoming divorce are attributable to the fact that Karen is the initiator and Bill is the noninitiator–that is, it is Karen, not Bill, who seeks the divorce. Dr. Levy recommends that Bill suspend all legal action for a few weeks while he processes his feelings about the divorce. She offers to refer him to a new therapist or to work with him herself.

Dr. Levy also helps Bill review the advice that he has received from his lawyer. She observes that even though lawyers are knowledgeable about divorce law, they do not fully comprehend or appreciate the emotional consequences of some of the tactics they routinely recommend. She encourages Bill to carefully consider the emotional implications of staying in the house with Karen and the children through a lengthy divorce, and also discusses the importance of understanding each other's need to build a new life.

Bill opts to continue therapy with Dr. Levy, since he already has a rapport with her and is reluctant to begin with someone new. During the next few weeks, he begins to regard his marriage in a different light. He acknowledges that, while Karen has been the one to make the decision to terminate the marriage, they have been drifting apart for a long time. His interests and hers have diverged, and he has been spending increasing amounts of time at the office to avoid facing a wife he has little in common with. He admits that his indignation is misplaced and might be self-defeating. At this point, Dr. Levy works with Bill to help him shift his focus to solving the problems of the future and to working on ways to ensure that all members of the family will thrive. Bill stops concentrating on how to win a struggle and begins looking at to how to recruit Karen's cooperation and work with her to find solutions.

COMMENTARY: Bill needs time to come to terms with his emotions, accept responsibility for his part in the progressive deterioration of the marriage, and acknowledge that the marriage is really ending. Once he has done so, he is in a position to begin looking toward the future instead of ruminating on the past or dwelling on Karen's faults. Dr. Levy's proactive intervention has enabled him to reach this important juncture.

The Role of the Counselor in Recommending Mediation

After several sessions, Dr. Levy brings up the subject of mediation, explaining that it is a way for Bill and Karen to negotiate a settlement that will be fair to both parties and will enable them to retain the ability to communicate with each other and work as a team in parenting. And although the couple will eventually use lawyers as advisors, the role of the lawyers would be limited to advice. He and Karen would therefore retain control of the process.

Bill is skeptical. He wonders if it is possible for his interests to be served or whether he might not make concessions he will regret later. Perhaps he really does need a lawyer to fight for him. Dr. Levy assures him that mediation is a process in which the interests of both parties are served. She recommends several mediators she had used in the past. Bill researches the mediators and reads up on mediation. His fears are somewhat allayed, and he suggests to Karen that they consider mediation.

Like Bill, Karen is initially skeptical. Wouldn't she be overpowered by Bill in the negotiation? Who would represent her interests? How would she know if the mediator would be fair? Bill pleads with her to discuss the matter with her own therapist as well as Dr. Levy.

Karen's counselor encourages her to at least have one meeting with the mediator and then decide if she wants to continue. The counselor emphasizes that mediation is completely voluntary and Karen has nothing to lose but an hour of her time. Karen also calls Dr. Levy, who assures her that mediation offers the best chance for an efficient and timely resolution of the divorce and the best chance of helping Bill to manage his feelings and negotiate fairly. Karen agrees to one meeting with the mediator.

COMMENTARY: Bill and Karen are both skeptical. Each is afraid that he or she will be taken advantage of, and neither has heard of mediation before. Both must override their preconceptions of how divorces are transacted and the advice of their family and friends, who think that they are "nuts" to try to work things out on their own.

Starting Mediation

Bill and Karen consult Mary Miles, a mediator who has been in practice for many years. Ms. Miles had originally been a conventional divorce lawyer but had become disillusioned with conventional law practice, a process that she felt caused much harm. Now she limits her practice to mediation.

Ms. Miles listens to the couple and then suggests that they should be able to resolve their issues in about 8–10 sessions. Karen likes Ms. Miles's calm manner and gets the impression that she understands not only the law but also how to handle people. She feels reassured that Bill will not be able to bully her and that mediation will be a fair process.

Ms. Miles asks each of them how they see the major issues. Karen says that she wants to go to law school and wants Bill to support her until she is able to establish a career, a process that will probably take 5–6 years. She also wants Bill to move out so that she can continue to live in the house with the children. Certainly she would like the children to see their father and to maintain a good relationship with him, but she feels she should be the primary parent because this has always been her role.

Bill wants to stay with the kids. He doesn't see why he should be the one forced to move out. All their savings are in the house, and if he moves out he will be unable to buy another house for 5 years. Owning a house is very important, as he spends his spare time in his garden and in his workshop and would be unable to have those things if he moves into an apartment. He also disagrees that Karen has to be the primary parent. After all, he has also been involved with the kids' lives, coaching their teams and helping them with their homework. He is as competent as Karen at cooking and taking care of the house and does not accept the assumption that Karen should remain the primary caregiver. Lastly, he feels strongly that Karen should get a teaching job to help out. Two households are more expensive than one, and they are already using up his entire salary just to run one household. How will they make it if Karen doesn't go to work? After all, it's not his problem that Karen wants to go to law school. She can go part-time and take out student loans. In the meantime, she needs to get a job.

Karen becomes angry. "You see, that just shows he's not really interested in helping me!" Bill starts an angry rebuttal, but Ms. Miles calms both of them. Then she requests individual meetings with each in the following week. All subsequent meetings will be joint, but she wants an opportunity to get to know each of them a little better. She invites Bill and Karen to talk to their respective therapists on an ongoing basis about the emotional ramifications of the legal and practical issues that are being worked out in the mediator's office. "These are separate but related processes," she says as the couple is leaving. "The most favorable outcome of mediation will be linked to your emotional ability to work together and carry out whatever is decided here."

COMMENTARY: In mediation, the couple's issues and opposing viewpoints are aired. Both Karen and Bill feel that the mediator has listened carefully and that each has been given the chance to speak his or her mind. While neither is completely convinced that the issues can be resolved this way, both are willing to give it another try. They feel comforted that mediation and therapy can work hand in hand and will strengthen and augment each other.

Individual Sessions

The following week Karen and Bill have their individual meetings with Ms. Miles. For the first part of the meeting, Ms. Miles just listens and occasionally probes. She encourages both clients to tell her everything on their minds about the divorce. Then she began to explore options. Why could the house not be sold so each could afford a less expensive house? How much equity is in the house, and what are townhouses and smaller houses selling for in the area? When Karen worries that a move would be too disruptive for the children, Ms. Miles points out that a move within the same town that does not involve change in schools or friends is not really very disruptive and that the children can manage it if their parents cooperate.

She asks Karen if she thinks the case can be amicably resolved if it means that Bill would have to live in an apartment. Karen acknowledges that it is unlikely and that some solution must be found to keep Bill in a house. The mediator also asks Karen why she believes it is her job to take care of the children. After all, Karen has shouldered that responsibility for 17 years. Now that the kids are more independent and she wants to pursue a new career, wouldn't it be fair to her to have Bill do more of the work so she can succeed in law school?

Karen has never thought of the issue in those terms. She has always believed mothers who "give up" custody of their kids are "bad mothers." If she lets Bill assume the primary role, wouldn't that mean that she is a bad mother? "Only if you insist on framing it that way," Ms. Miles responds. "I'm sure you and Bill can work out a shared parenting agreement that shifts more of the responsibility to him but keeps you in an important close role with the children." Karen agrees to think about it.

When Ms. Miles meets with Bill, he expresses two concerns. He does not want to live in an apartment, and he does not want to pay long-term alimony. This is why he has been so insistent about Karen getting a job immediately. Ms. Miles asks Bill to analyze how much money Karen would earn as a teacher over the next 10 years and then compare that to what Karen would earn if she went to law school for the next 3 years and then worked as a lawyer in a firm for the subsequent 7 years. Bill does some calculations and discovers that Karen's total income would actually be considerably higher if she went to law school. She would be better able to help with the cost of tuition that would become almost crushing with all three children in college at the same time. Bill agrees to reconsider the subject with this new angle in mind.

COMMENTARY: The mediator has given the couple a private and safe forum in which each was able to articulate his or her real concerns and objectives. Having done so, she lays out the various options under consideration and explores how to best meet their objectives. Bill and Karen feel validated and understood and are able to reevaluate the positions that each has held firmly and realize that compromise might be possible.

Agreements Reached during Mediation

Over the next few meetings, Bill and Karen work out their settlement. They refinance the house to get enough equity out for a down payment on a townhouse for Karen. In 2 years the present house will be sold and the equity divided so Bill can buy a smaller house. Bill agrees to pay alimony to Karen until she finishes law school and for 1 year after that if she needs it. The children will continue to spend most of their time in the house with Bill but will spend weekends and any other time they want with Karen. The couple decide to call their arrangement joint custody even though the children live primarily with Bill. For Karen, being formally designated as anything less than an equal parent was too difficult, and Bill agreed to the joint custody designation to make Karen comfortable. They know that finances will be tight, but with the help of student loans they believe they can make it. These agreements become the settlement for their divorce.

COMMENTARY: Both Bill and Karen have had to alter their original scenarios of what their divorce would look like. But each feels they have reached a viable and reasonable solution.

Epilogue

Five years later, the family is doing well. The oldest child is graduating from college this year, and both younger children are thriving. All three have gone to state colleges, and the family was able to manage the financial strain. Karen graduated from law school this year and is starting as an associate in a major law firm. Her first-year salary is twice what she would have been earning as a teacher. She is happy in her new career. Nothing came of her relationship with Craig, but she did meet a man during her last year of law school, and they are well on their way to a long-term relationship.

Bill remarried 2 years ago and is quite happy in his new life. Bill and Karen are not friends, but neither are they hostile. They have been able to cooperate around the children, and both regard the children's success with pride. The children like Bill's new wife and the man Karen is dating.

COMPARING THE OUTCOMES

Let's compare the outcomes of these two cases in light of the six components of a good divorce outlined earlier in Sidebar 2.1.

1. Emotional Disengagement

People divorce in order to begin new lives and usually hope these new lives will involve new mates. One cannot achieve a successful new relationship without ending the prior one. Many couples on the cusp of divorce express the desire to come out of the process as friends. That is not likely. It is extremely difficult to go from an intimate relationship to a platonic friendship, and it is unlikely that a friendship can survive all the pain necessarily attendant to a divorce. But it is possible to avoid coming out of the divorce with an active enemy. If one spouse emerges feeling humiliated and poorly treated, he or she may never be able to let go of powerful feelings of anger and betrayal. There is a big difference between remembering that you once had feelings of intense anger, and actually regurgitating and reexperiencing those feelings. It is possible for people who have had decent divorces to get on with their lives so that the feelings toward their ex-spouses, both positive and negative, become progressively weaker and in time play no part in a new life. There may be some fond memories, and there may be troubled memories. But what is important is that the feelings for the ex-spouse are no longer compelling and are no longer able to mobilize the person's emotions.

Bad divorce is characterized by just the opposite. One or both spouses cannot let go and must stay connected with the other. This process is reinforced by remaining in continuous conflict that prolongs the divorce and makes conflict a never-ending state of affairs. Some couples become chronic litigants, dragging each other back to court year after year in order to win in the latest squabble. They may win some battles, but ultimately they lose the war. Because they are never able to fully disengage, they are never able to acquire the necessary distance and indifference that are prerequisite to really starting over. The ongoing conflict affects all aspects of the divorced family's life. Visitation with children is never smooth. Fathers show up late or cancel at the last minute, and mothers interfere with and sabotage the father's time with the children. Chronic litigants often infect each other's new marriages, and new spouses give up because life is a perpetual battle with the former spouse. The endless cycle of provocation and litigation poisons the parents' ability to cooperate for the benefit of the children, and the children often develop depression or other psychological symptoms as a result. The children's problems, in turn, affect the parents' ability to lead independent lives, as they become increasingly entangled in the challenges posed by needy or poorly behaved children.

In our two case studies, Dick and Tammy experience chronic conflict. Because each feels cheated and humiliated by the other, they are having a hard time completing the divorce and working through the harsh emotions that go along with it. Each has trouble letting the other live in peace, and as a consequence neither is thriving. Their children are showing the effects of the strain, and their demands are increasing. By contrast, Bill and Karen have managed to get through their divorce with their civility and sense of self-respect intact. They are doing well and are emotionally free of each other. Their children, likewise, are thriving. They have a good divorce.

2. Rebuilding Lives

In my experience, the 5-year juncture after a divorce is an important benchmark in assessing whether a couple has been successful in rebuilding their lives. Even a good divorce is characterized by social losses associated with the change. Friends of the divorced couple tend to drop away. Although some may manage to maintain a relationship with both divorced partners, many end up choosing only one of the partners with whom to continue social contact. Others shy away from both partners. Newly single people often report surprise that long-term friends seem to avoid them or just fail to include them. The family of each divorced partner generally pulls away from the former in-law, even though some try to maintain a cordial relationship for the benefit of the children. So, for many divorced people, particularly men, loneliness is a common result of divorce. Women tend to have more close women friends with whom they exchange intimacies. Men appear less likely to have intimate male friends.

Church membership also may not represent a resource for divorcing people. Only recently have churches, synagogues, and other faith communities developed ministries for their divorced couples, and there are still no formal or ritualistic events for reintegrating the divorced couple as single members of the congregation. As a result, many divorced people end up leaving their churches or temples—especially if the ex-spouse remains affiliated. Starting over in a new church just poses one more hurdle to overcome, another arena in which there is a new beginning to be faced and navigated.

So, most newly divorced people need to consciously rebuild their social lives. Eventually, they reach a point where they are ready to look for another potential mate. The initiator of the divorce typically does this first and indeed may have begun to clandestinely date others even before announcing the decision to divorce. The noninitiator may need more time before he or she is ready to date. For most people, dating does not bring pleasure but rather is fraught with insecurity and awkwardness. An entire singles and dating industry has grown up to serve this population. (In a later chapter we will delve into more detail about how to establish a substantive fulfilling life after divorce.)

Most people succeed in rebuilding. About 80% of men are remarried within 2 years of divorce, and about 75% of women remarry within 10 years. About 55–60% of those remarriages will end in divorce.[2] There are some people who never regain a social footing. In my experience, these are the people who had the worst divorces. Some come out of the divorce so bitter that they are unable to trust anyone enough to rebuild a successful new relationship. Others have created so much economic disarray that they just can't get themselves reorganized, and end up marginal and virtually incapacitated. Still others have so damaged their children that they are unable to find another potential mate willing to live through the chaos generated by the would-be stepchildren.

In many ways, the ones who had the easiest, least conflict-ridden, divorces adjust better and rebuild with greater success. It is easier to create second families when the children of the first marriage are not a source of perpetual disruption. It is easier to court and be courted when you have adequate amounts of time away from your children. Finally, it is difficult to build a new relationship when you are still riveted to the first. Prolonged litigation and conflict that continues after the divorce is over distract people from a new relationship and leave them without the emotional energy to forge a successful connection to someone new.

Dick and Tammy illustrate what happens when the divorce is not resolved well. They are unable to free themselves from the consequences of the way in which their divorce was managed. The maladaptation of their children prevents Tammy from finding someone new and causes difficulties in Dick's second marriage. It is not uncommon that the foundation of the second divorce is laid brick by brick during the first. Dick and Tammy will have to free themselves of each other and release their anger and bitterness before they will be able to build successful new lives. Bill and Karen, on the other hand, have emotional and practical closure regarding their relationship and divorce and are able to move on, unimpeded.

3. Both Think the Agreement Is Fair

When Dick and Tammy went to court, they came away with a settlement agreement, a fact that would suggest that both agreed to the

[2]Bramlett, M. D., & Mosher, W. D. (2001). *First marriage dissolution, divorce, and remarriage: United States*. Advanced data from Vitaland Health Statistics, No. 323. Hyattsville, MD: National Center for Health Statistics.

terms. Actually, although most divorces are eventually resolved by a negotiated agreement, in about half of those cases the couple is back in court within 2 years continuing the fight over the children and support. With a 50% failure rate, there must be something essentially defective in those settlement agreements and the process that produces them.

Recall how Dick and Tammy received their settlement. They sat passively in the courtroom hallway while their lawyers met with the judge behind closed doors and "worked it out." Neither party participated in creating the agreement, and both felt it had been imposed on them. So, neither had any commitment to living in accordance with the agreement. As a result, they remain locked in continuing conflict and unable to finish with the divorce or with each other.

By contrast, Karen and Bill negotiated directly without the intervention of a coercive court system. They took all the time they needed to negotiate and explore options and to be creative about using their resources to attend to the needs of the entire family. Because they crafted their settlement largely by themselves, they accept ownership and are prepared to live by it. And because they each think it is fair, they are able to move on and successfully disconnect from each other.

4. Ability to Cooperate as Parents

One of the most important indicators of a good divorce is the emergence between the former spouses of a working partnership as parents. Children need both parents, and they need both parents to have functioning homes in which the children feel comfortable physically and emotionally. They also need parents who are not riveted by quarreling and can provide nurturing, guidance, and discipline. Many divorcing parents have to acquire a new model for communication, because their old patterns based on friendship and mutual affection are no longer applicable. I suggest to divorcing clients that they address each other as they would a colleague or customer. Such communication is characterized by respect and cordiality and even occasional warmth, but does not include intimacy. There is a job to be done, and another human being is required as a collaborator in that job. Intimate observations or angry responses that would be inappropriate in business are also inappropriate between divorced parents. The couple has a single common interest–the children–and each expects the other's best effort in that area. But their communication reflects their awareness that they have no emotional claim on each other.

A civil working partnership is difficult to achieve when people are in a state of active rage with each other or when the children have been psychologically damaged by the divorce and are acting out as a result. The emotional dysfunction that flows from a bad divorce makes it unlikely that people can achieve the cooperation a parental partnership requires. Dick and Tammy have been unable to achieve this partnership, but Karen and Bill have succeeded in doing so.

5. Children Are Comfortable in Each Household

The adjustment to divorce is a long-term proposition, often taking several years. Long-term adjustment begins with several important factors that have taken place during the divorce. First, neither parent has recruited the children as allies against the other. Rather, each parent has made clear to the children that they have played no role in the disputes between the parents and has encouraged the children to like and respect the other parent. Each has promoted the other parent as loving and competent, and neither has used the children to sabotage the other parent. Finally, each parent has encouraged the children to like or at least respect the new spouse or partner of the other parent. Each child feels that he or she has each parent's consent to be comfortable in the other's household.

By this standard, Dick and Tammy have failed, while Bill and Karen have succeeded. Because Dick and Tammy have been unable to finish their divorce with a mutual sense of justice, neither can support the other as a parent. Their continual return to court to fight over children and money continues to alienate the children and to disrupt their lives. Tammy has spoken negatively about Dick's new wife and has undermined Dick's parenting skills. Bill and Karen, on the other hand, are able to cooperate as parents. They succeed in moving on to new lives and integrate the children without continuing hostility and bitterness.

6. The Former Spouses Are Able to Resolve Disputes Themselves

The lives of divorced people do not remain static. If things go well for each of the former spouses, their lives will evolve and change as they build new relationships and adapt to living in separate households. New jobs and new mates may require relocation. Layoffs and promotions will change economic circumstances. Health problems may necessitate adjustments in routine and in finances. And children change as they get older. Their social patterns change, their preferences change, they mature, start dating, driving, and developing new hobbies and interests. Divorced parents with children usually learn that their support and parenting arrangements may need to be modified as their children grow older. The important question is whether the parties are able to resolve issues of change as they arise and how they will manage when they don't agree about what to do.

I regard the ability to resolve differences amicably and constructively to be the ultimate indicator of a good divorce. Dick and Tammy are unable to let go of their conflict and, so, unable to resolve any disputes without going to court. They will be "married" to each other through conflict as long as they have dependent children, and that conflict will continually contaminate their lives. Bill and Karen, on the other hand, are able to resolve differences when they arise. So, disputes are disposed of quickly, meaning each may move on. I always encourage couples whose divorces I mediate to incorporate mediation clauses into their separation agreements. The mediation clause creates an obligation to return to mediation whenever an issue arises that they cannot resolve by themselves. In most cases this keeps them out of court and allows them to find solutions to their problems–usually in a single hour-long session. Although it would be better if they could resolve their disputes without any help, the presence of the mediation clause usually prevents an issue from festering and helps couples to adapt to change.

ACHIEVING A GOOD DIVORCE

Understanding is key to mastering the therapeutic skills necessary to achieve the goal of a good divorce. By "understanding," I mean several things: (1) an understanding of the legal procedures that couples must go through in order to be called "divorced"; (2) an understanding of the legal culture within which the laws and procedures of divorce are enacted, and the mindset of the lawyers who are entrusted with transacting the divorce process; (3) an understanding of the psychology of divorcing couples and the emotional issues they confront and that they must overcome; and (4) an understanding of the variety of practical decisions they must make and how these decisions affect the outcome of the divorce. The chapters that follow elaborate on these essential areas of knowledge.

3 Managing the Decision to Divorce

Although no-fault divorce has been around for 30 years, the psyches of divorcing couples have not always caught up with the trend. Many couples continue to attack each other using the court system to deny responsibility for the failure of the marriage, heap blame on the other, and then use all this to argue that the dislocations of the divorce should fall disproportionately on the other "guilty" spouse. Here is where the interactivity of the legal process and emotional process is seen most clearly. Despite no-fault divorce, what the legal system does best is to find fault. After all, this is what it was designed for, and in the absence of a very clear mandate to the contrary, it reverts quickly to its faultfinding role. So, it is ready-made for the spouse who feels so injured by the bad behavior of the other that he or she wants revenge and vindication.

The process begins with the decision to divorce. Unless a couple has been counseled to the point of divorce, it is easy for one or both to explain the entire marital failure in terms of the bad acts of the other. Sins of omission–failure to communicate, failure to do one's share or contribute one's share, failure to be affectionate or supportive or caring–are catalogued and reviewed. Sins of commission–infidelity, indifference, slovenly ways, meanness, selfishness–are also reviewed and hurled as accusations at the other.

The focus on the actions and/or inactions of the other spouse as the "cause" of the divorce allows the client to avoid thoughts about his or her own contribution to the marriage's demise. The focus on the court as the place to get justice feeds the fantasy that an authoritative source will uphold one's version of reality and vindicate one while punishing the spouse. Finally, the circle is completed by the fantasy that in meting out justice the court will put a disproportionate share of the dislocation of divorce on the other spouse while allowing your client to go forward unscathed. When both spouses get caught up in this system, divorces become truly poisonous.

Thus, the decision to divorce is arguably the most critical time in a divorce. This stage occurs during the month or two immediately following the announcement by one spouse to the other that he or she wants to end the marriage. There is a considerable gap in the psychological readiness of the initiator versus the noninitiator to accept the myriad changes associated with divorce. This can become the source of intense hostility and recrimination. Here is where the therapist can begin to make a significant difference in determining whether the divorce will be peaceful or acrimonious.

For most people, divorce is both a crisis and a first-time experience. Even for those ending second marriages, divorce is traumatic, and the first divorce seldom provides a workable model for the second. So, there is usually precious little of the knowledge needed to manage the process well. First off, few people understand the law or the legal process. Moreover, few people–and particularly the noninitiators–have thought through the practical realities of divorce. In the absence of knowledge, they have to rely on what they *think* they know, combined with whatever information they glean from other people. The "Greek chorus" of family, friends, and acquaintances usually provides incomplete, incorrect, and downright damaging guidance. The typical result is a proliferation of bad decisions based on immediate reactions and feelings rather than a dispassionate appreciation of one's long-term interests. The therapist's role is to provide accurate and relevant information and to help the client manage the emotions that accompany the decision to divorce.

We will look at two different scenarios: when the client is the initiator of the divorce and when the client is the noninitiator.

COUNSELING THE INITIATOR

The person who initiates the divorce starts out in control of the process. The role of the therapist is to educate the client about how to manage the initial stage, how to break the news to the other spouse, and how to recruit the other spouse to a collaborative and cooperative divorce. In most cases, if the client does not get this instruction from the therapist, he or she is unlikely to get it anywhere else. An initiator must understand several important issues.

Clarity and Certainty about the Decision

By the time the initiator has decided to divorce, we would hope that he or she has had ample opportunity to establish that the marriage is really over. My criterion for this decision is clarity on the part of the initiator that there is nothing that the other spouse can do or say that will lead to a change of heart. It is important to review this with the client, even if he or she has been in therapy and has been contemplating divorce for some time. On too many occasions I have seen a person use the announcement of the divorce as a last-ditch attempt to induce some desired behavioral change in the other spouse. He or she would really like to avoid the divorce but is hoping to shock the other into paying attention. I think this approach is a bad idea, because this ploy, in itself, does damage to the relationship. I recently worked with a couple in which the wife initiated the divorce. After she told her husband, she was shocked when he embraced the decision. As it turned out, she was only using the announcement of the divorce as a gesture to get him to agree to counseling. She really did not want the divorce and was bitter when he jumped at the suggestion. Some initiators like the idea of "trying out" what it might be like to announce the intention to divorce to gauge the spouse's reaction, but they are still ambivalent. Clearly, nothing should be said about the decision until the client has tried everything else and is now completely certain that the marriage must end.

Understanding the Initiator/Noninitiator Dimension

The initiator must understand the difference between his or her psychological readiness for the divorce and that of the spouse. Initiators have to be armed with realistic expectations of the emotional needs of the other spouse so that the spouse is given sufficient time to come to grips with the decision. In many cases, the spouse will not be totally surprised, because the couple has likely been having problems for years. In other cases, the spouse will be thunderstruck and cast into emotional disarray. Clients should be coached on not only how to break the news but also on how to manage the reaction of the other partner. I will talk more about that later. The therapist should review with the client the fact that the divorce will require many changes in the organization and finances of the family. While the initiator has had the time necessary to reconcile him- or herself to the losses that accompany divorce, the noninitiators has not had this opportunity. For the initiator, losses are offset by gains. For the noninitiator, there are only losses. So, the initiator must understand that it may take some time before the spouse can respond and begin productive discussions about how the separation and divorce should be managed.

Once the decision has been announced, initiators are often eager to get things under way. Thus, a wife who initiates a divorce may be eager to see her husband move out of the house, or a husband who initiates it may be eager to get the house sold so that he and his wife can divide the proceeds. But in each of these cases the noninitiator is not ready to have such discussions, and prematurely broaching such topics is likely to frighten the other party and induce him or her to seek rescue in a lawyer's office. The other consequence of bad timing here is that is gives the noninitiator the impression that the initiating spouse is totally insensitive to his or her needs, thus engendering bad faith early in the divorce process. So, proper timing is a special consideration that should be discussed at length early on.

Telling the Spouse

Here are some principles to teach the initiator about telling the spouse of the decision to divorce.

Be Gentle

The tone to be used is similar to the tone one would use to tell a person that a loved one has died. This requires choosing a time when both have privacy and are not in the middle of a confrontation.

> "Marty, I have some difficult news that I know you will find upsetting. I have decided that we need to divorce."

Be Clear

The message has to include the fact that the decision is irrevocable and that nothing can induce a change of heart.

> "I have been thinking about this for a long time, and although I know it will be hard for all of us for a while, I am sure that it is the right decision and I am clear that this is necessary. I don't think there is anything that either of us can do to fix the marriage, and I believe this is the only thing to do."

Letting the spouse know that the decision is firm cannot be stressed enough. One problem that I see repeatedly is the illusion of "temporary separation" as a way to ease the blow of divorce. Here, the initiator says something like this: "We have been having trouble for so long that the only thing that will help is for us to separate for a while just to have some peace and some space and be able to think clearly. Maybe after we do that, we will figure out what we really want and maybe be able to get back together again." The implication is that the separation may lead to reconciliation and that the decision to end the marriage can be altered.

Sometimes when the initiator says this she (or he) may really believe that this is true. She knows the marriage cannot go on with the status quo. She knows it is not working and does not know how to fix it. Her feelings for her spouse are predominantly negative, and she believes that it would be a great relief if he would move out. And the relief that would bring is more important and more urgent than the absolute definition of whether the marriage is really over. Or, she may really believe that living apart will give everyone a chance to sort out emotions and make the best decisions. But, in my experience, this ploy is used more often as a way to ease the blow and to get the spouse out of the house without having to deal with the confrontation that will come if she says very decisively that the marriage is over. The idea is to separate under the guise of "temporary separation" and then just not get back together. The news about the divorce can be transmitted after the couple has been separated for 2–6 months. This way, when the other spouse reacts angrily, he is already out of the house.

From what I have seen, "temporary separation" is seldom a good idea. Very few marriages are improved by separation. If there is enough left of the marriage to repair it and save it, people should stay together and work on the marriage. In my experience, using temporary separation as a guise invariably results in greater anger later when the noninitiating spouse—who has been led to think that the marriage might resume—realizes that there was never any real intention to resume the marriage. He or she feels duped and is reluctant to trust the other thereafter.

I frequently see couples that come for mediation with one spouse presenting the goal as being a temporary separation. A few questions usually suffice to enable the real intention to surface. The most telling is the question of whether the spouses are free to date during the separation. On a few occasions, both spouses reply in the negative and state that they will remain faithful during this period. But more commonly, the initiator will state something to the effect that "Of course, we should be free to date others. How else will we be able to tell if we really want the marriage to resume?" So, then I ask whether dating would include the right to have sex with others. If the initiator says that yes, they should be free to have sex with others, the other spouse almost always catches on and concludes that the real subject under discussion is divorce. But it is much better to have it resolved this way than to separate under false pretenses and have the noninitiating spouse discover that the initiator is sleeping with someone else. So, to clarify, I would add honesty as an approach to telling the noninitiator about the divorce. The therapist may be involved here as either an individual therapist or a couple therapist. A couples therapist might well have a discussion with the couple similar to that described above. But an individual therapist will also be able to explain, at least to one party, that temporary separation is not a great idea.

Provide Reassurance

The initiator must reassure his (or her) spouse that, although the marriage is over, he will do everything he can to be fair and gentle. For example, assume for this illustration that the initiator is a husband. He might deliver the news of his decision to divorce in the following way:

> "I know this is very painful and I am very sorry to do this, but I am at my wits' end and just can't see an alternative. I don't have the feelings that are necessary to make it work. There is too much distance between us to overcome. The marriage is over. I am worried about the children, and I am concerned for you. The marriage has to end, but I will do everything I can to do it decently and fairly."

The initiator should anticipate an angry response and be warned not to defend himself. When a person does not defend, an attack ceases. His wife could well say something like this:

> "How can you do such a rotten thing to me and the kids? What kind of heartless bastard are you that you would leave us like this? I'm going to find the meanest lawyer I can get, and I'm going to take you for everything I can!"

The initiator should be coached to respond:

> "I know that this is upsetting and very painful, and I am going to do my best to be fair. We can talk about it again later if you wish, and I will do my best to help you understand why I believe that this is necessary."

The essence of this dialogue may have to be repeated several times until the angry response is diffused.

Use Neutral Language and Avoid Imputing Fault and Blame

It can be tempting to shift the responsibility for the failure of the marriage onto the other spouse or to list the spouse's wrongdoings that have led up to the decision. This is a mistake, and clients should be counseled away from such an approach.

> "I have been in pain for a long time about our marriage and no longer believe we can fix it. I'm not blaming you. I know you have done your best and I have done my best. But it just doesn't work and it has to end."

Give the Noninitiator Time to Absorb the News

The initiator should say that she will wait as long as necessary and that she has no intention of doing anything until her spouse has had time to think and is ready to talk.

> "I know that this is difficult for you, and I want you to know that I am not doing anything with lawyers and that I will wait until you are ready to talk so we can figure out how to do this as decently as we can."

The purpose of this coaching is to give the client the opportunity to practice how he or she will tell the spouse and to avoid saying things reflexively that will be regretted later. This is a difficult task for most people, because they feel guilty about imposing pain on someone else, they are worried about the children, and they are worried about causing a scene replete with anger, recrimination, and tears. The client may also be angry with the spouse and see this as an opportunity to say angry things. But it is most important for the client to understand that this is the opening scene in a script that has not yet been written and that it will set the tone for the entire divorce to come.

COACHING THE NONINITIATOR

If you are the therapist for the noninitiator, your initial task is helping him or her to respond appropriately after the initiator has broken the news. Here you don't have the opportunity to plan the initial interaction, and you have to respond depending on how the initial discussion between the spouses played out. If the client was not expecting this news or if the initial discussion was acrimonious, you have a more difficult time than if it was handled well and gently. So, your first task may be to calm the client down enough to begin analyzing the situation. What is most undesirable is for the client to engage in precipitous action. There is no reason to run to a lawyer, although a consultation with a lawyer will be appropriate in time. In fact, there is no need to do anything in particular in the immediate aftermath of the initial discussion about divorce. The client needs some time to reflect and to get control of him- or herself and the situation before he or she does anything.

Accepting the Divorce

Depending on where the client is on the continuum of acceptance, the initial discussion will be about whether the divorce is real. First, is the other spouse serious, and is the situation reversible? Except in the unusual case in which the other spouse is using the threat of divorce as a gesture, my experience suggests that by the time one spouse actually says, "I want a divorce," the marriage is dead. The noninitiator may already know that to be the truth but has been reluctant or too frightened to admit it.

> "Well, I guess it was inevitable. We've been having problems for years and have been to marriage counseling more times than I can count. I have tried everything I know, but nothing works. We just can't get on the same wavelength, and things have been getting worse all the time."

When the client says something similar to this, you know that the divorce is more or less mutual and that it will not be long before this client is ready to begin the work of planning the separation.

But the client may also be completely thunderstruck by the news from the other spouse.

> "I was caught totally off guard by Marie's announcement last night. I thought we were getting along just fine. Sure, we have our troubles, just like anyone else, but nothing to warrant divorce. I don't understand this at all."

This is the client who will require the most work. He will need to explore how he missed so many cues that he never saw the divorce coming. The very fact that he and his wife are so out of sync may be the first thing you discuss as an indicator that something is wrong. You will need to help him investigate the marital history and try to figure out what was really going on that he missed. What has his spouse been saying about her needs? What has she been asking of him that he has been ignoring? What distress calls has he missed? Not only will he require a lot of work to get ready to separate; he will require much work just understanding the marriage. This is a client who would benefit from divorce therapy with his spouse–not to reconcile but to get a better understanding about why the marriage is ending. If he can convince the initiating spouse to enter into this process, divorce therapy is a much better way to investigate the divorce than having the two try to have these discussions alone. If they try it without a therapist to moderate, there is too much likelihood that the conversation will deteriorate into blaming and recrimination, with more heat than light as the result.

Avoiding Blaming the Initiator

Rather than accept any responsibility for the demise of the marriage, a noninitiator who is surprised by news of the divorce typically goes on a search for explanations that will find the other spouse at fault for the marital breakup.

> "I have tried but she has not. She is just immature and thinks life can be some fairy tale with never-ending passion and living happily ever after. She has never been willing to do the hard parts of a marriage. She has always been selfish, and this is just another example of that. She doesn't give a damn about the kids or me; all she cares about is her own wants. I wonder if she has a boyfriend. Maybe I should hire a private detective."

Unless you assume that your client is among the few people who have contributed nothing to the failure of the marriage, you will do him a favor by deflecting him from this path.

Avoiding the Victim Role

For the noninitiator, managing anger when rejected is a difficult but crucial task at the outset of the divorce. Anger can be a shuck for one's own responsibility. When you get angry with someone, you are able to focus all your hurt feelings on the behavior of that person. If it's her fault, it's easy to believe it isn't your fault. The more intense and elaborate your own anger, the less you have to feel difficult feelings about your own actions. The noninitiator who blames the initiator avoids responsibility and slides into the role of the victim.

> "I didn't do anything wrong. I am completely innocent and am therefore being victimized by the bad behavior of my wife. She is being selfish (childish, irresponsible, mean, etc.). She has abandoned me (and the kids), she is having an affair and is betraying me, she has led me on all these years and never really loved me, she has used me all this time and now that she doesn't need me is dumping me. But I have done nothing wrong. She is doing everything wrong. She is a bad person. I am the victim. She should be punished."

The victim often engages in a plaintive song of woe as he recounts and lists all the terrible things the other spouse has done and all the character deficits of the other. Soon the story gets ever more elaborate. Because all the wrong rests with the other, because the client is innocent and the other is guilty, because the client is the victim, the spouse must be the villain. Victims need villains, and villains should be punished. In the context of divorce, villains should be punished by having to accept responsibility for all the nasty consequences of divorce. That is, all those unpleasant changes that divorce requires should be heaped on the villainous spouse.

> "Why should I suffer? Why should the kids suffer? My spouse has brought this about–so, let her pay. Let her move out and leave the kids and me in the house. Let her get a job and support herself and maybe even pay me child support. I have struggled all these years to save some money and build a pension account. Let her go build her own accounts and leave mine alone. She ought to get nothing, because she deserves nothing."

There are three problems with the victim's posture. First, it helps to reinforce the illusion that someday the victim will get vindicated and the other will get punished. But the judicial system doesn't do this very well, as we shall see. And then there is the second problem. If we want to punish the other spouse for wrongdoing, the only available forum is the courts, and that means a long process of litigation and all the emotional and financial exhaustion it produces. The only punishment inflicted is that the couple will have an awful divorce and that both will suffer. The villain might be left financially broken, but so will the victim. The relationship of both with the children will also be damaged. The solace won by embracing the victim's role will be very temporary.

Lastly, when a client assumes the role of victim, he or she misses the opportunity for growth and learning that is derived from assuming one's appropriate share of the responsibility for either the divorce or the adjustment to divorce. Helping the client sort this out is one of the greatest services that the therapist can provide.

Victims and Children

When one parent assumes the victim's role, the impact on the children can be devastating. The victim parent behaves so pathetically that the children feel that they have to rescue that parent. They take it upon themselves to comfort and reassure him. And as the victimized parent confides in the child and seeks comfort, he recruits the child to share his anger at the mother who is initiating the divorce.

> "Mommy is breaking up the family. She wants to leave you and me."

Assuming that this ploy is successful–and it frequently is–the child comes to the rescue and becomes angry with the other parent. Because the child is now taking care of the victimized parent and is alienated from the other parent, he or she has effectively just lost both parents. During the onset of divorce, children are understandably needy and require extra attention and nurturing by both parents. In this scenario the child becomes an emotional orphan and, instead of being cared for by parents, finds him- or herself being the caregiver. The long-term results are very poor.

A second version of the victim mentality scenario occurs when the noninitiator extends the "poor me" attitude to a "poor children" attitude and uses this line of reasoning to launch a custody battle, ostensibly in the best interests of the children. The majority of custody fights I have seen involve men whose wives have initiated the divorce and who are holding on to the kids in the hope of also holding on to the house and the familiar structure of their lives.

> "You want this divorce–so, why don't you move out and leave me and the kids here. Why should all our lives be disrupted just because you decide to break your vows and have a second adolescence?"

This sentiment often then leads to an attempt to portray the wife as a poor mother and to convince everyone that the children would be better off in the care of their father. This portrait of the mother often gets painted when she is leaving the marriage for another man, and it is tempting to argue that her immoral behavior in the affair proves she is unfit to be the primary parent. When men are feeling rejected, when their egos are in tatters and their sense of identity as father and husband is suddenly shattered, it is easy for them to fall into self-deluding beliefs as a way to seek solace for the pain. It is also easy for the man to assume a pose as protector of the children, when he is really trying to minimize the dislocation the divorce will bring to his life. If they believe that the wife should move out of the house, it also means they will not have to move. If they believe that the children should stay with them, it means they will not have to cope with the painful feelings that living apart from the children will bring. The more of one's old life that can be preserved—the more one can shift the dislocation of divorce to the wife—the less one has to change.

Avoiding Appeals for Reconciliation

Most divorces involve at least one attempt at reconciliation. Typically, the noninitiator appeals to the initiator to try to restore the marriage one last time. The initiator, feeling guilty and wishing to appease the noninitiator, agrees, albeit reluctantly. But the reconciliation seldom works, because the marriage is already too damaged. In my experience, people tend to emerge from the failed reconciliation attempt angrier than when they started. Commonly, the noninitiator accuses the initiator of not trying hard enough and of leading him or her on.

The decision to seek reconciliation should be the subject of some hard questions from the therapist. What is left to work on? What will be different this time? What behaviors does each expect of the other that will be different than the marriage to date? Does the initiator still have the requisite level of commitment and affection necessary for the marriage to work? Or, is the initiator just appeasing the noninitiator? Although it is not the therapist's role to dissuade the couple from an attempt at reconciliation, it is appropriate for the therapist to pose the questions that, when answered, might save the client another round of disillusionment.

What the Noninitiator Needs from the Initiator

Your client needs to be coached to ask his or her spouse to accommodate his or her reasonable emotional needs. There are seven requests that are relevant here.

Time to Absorb the News

The noninitiator needs reasonable time to absorb the news and the implications of the divorce before he or she has to act. It may be a few weeks or it may be a few months. But she should not be flooded with a rash of things to do in anticipation of the divorce. She should not have to make any changes until she has had time to think through the divorce and to begin to accept that the marriage is over. There are many issues in which the therapist can be of assistance, but therapeutic intervention requires ample time to explore the emotional and practical ramifications of the initiator's announcement. So, your client has to tell the spouse that time is required. But, at the same time, the client has to acknowledge the legitimate needs of the initiator.

> "I understand that you have made the decision to divorce, and I accept that we will have to do that. You have had the time you need to come to terms with the divorce; now I need some time as well. I am not trying to cause delay, but I am sure this will go faster in the end if you can wait a few months while I figure this out."

The Right Time for Public Disclosure

The noninitiator needs reasonable time before other people are told, with the exception of the few confidants that he or she has probably confided in anyhow. The couple does not need superficial acquaintances or strangers asking about the divorce until both parties are ready to talk about it. The noninitiator may initially feel humiliated and embarrassed by the news. Many people still regard divorce as something shameful. A noninitiator may regard divorce as a personal failure in the eyes of the community and, at least in the beginning, may not want others to know and may not want to have to talk about it with well-meaning friends or acquaintances. The spouses can agree when they will make the divorce "public." Some realism is required here, and it may not be realistic to keep the secret for months and months; but a decent interval can be negotiated to allow the noninitiator to get used to the idea before having to deal with the response of the larger community. It is easy for us professionals to forget that many people, particularly those who are active in their churches, synagogues, or other places of worship, may find the public revelation of divorce extremely troubling. But in some cases it may be wise to tell people closely involved with the children and whose confidentiality is trustworthy, such as the school guidance counselor, if the children seem to be aware that something is going on.

Avoiding Premature Negotiation

Your client should request that the initiator refrain from pressing to negotiate or make important decisions about the divorce until he or she has had time to think about it. Initiators are often eager to resolve issues related to children, money, and property so that they can start their new lives. They want to remove the ambiguity of the situation as fast as possible and may tend to press for resolution well before the other spouse is ready. So, the noninitiator has to be clear that he or she is not ready now but will get ready as soon as possible. If the other spouse insists, your client can politely decline to participate.

> "I know you are eager to resolve these things, but I am not ready and am asking you to wait until I am. I promise to be ready as soon as I can."

This is a good time to begin coaching the client on the use of neutral language so your client can express needs without personally attacking the other spouse and inflaming the situation.

Telling the Children

Children should not be told about the divorce until both spouses are ready for the discussion. So, it is reasonable for the noninitiator to ask the spouse to agree that nothing be said to the children until the couple is ready to tell them jointly. This is another reason not to make the divorce public before the couple is ready to discuss it. There is nothing worse for children than hearing about the divorce from other people. Telling the children is a searing experience for most people, and the noninitiator must be ready before he or she is asked to have that discussion with the children.

Maintaining a Cordial Atmosphere

It is easy in the heat of the early stages of divorce for communication in the household to become rancorous. But when this happens, it makes it much harder on everyone to get through the process intact. The noninitiator needs to be coached that this is not the time for a stream of angry recriminations directed toward the spouse, because it only evokes reciprocal recrimination precisely at the time when your client most needs peace. It is desirable that the noninitiating client tell the initiator that he or she will work very hard to be civil and polite and to request that the other spouse behave that way as well. All this is counterintuitive for the client, so it may take some repetition before the client accepts the wisdom of this strategy. Most clients are able to succeed most of the time, but occasional outbreaks are not uncommon. The therapist can continue to support and counsel civility so that escalation of hostilities does not occur.

Divorce Counseling

It is not uncommon for the noninitiator to feel that he or she does not understand why the other is seeking a divorce.

> "I don't understand why you are doing this. Sure we had some troubles, but I never dreamed you were thinking about divorce. Please explain it to me–I just don't get it."

For many noninitiators, the unresolved reasons for the divorce can slow down the process of acceptance and lead to a refusal to accept the divorce. If this goes on long enough, the initiator gets angry and initiates litigation just to force the issue.

Divorce counseling, in which the couple has a few sessions with a couples counselor to talk about the reasons for the divorce, can be very helpful in these situations. Each spouse gets assistance in being heard and understood by the other. Because it makes acceptance easier for the noninitiator, divorce counseling serves the interest of both spouses. Your client needs to be coached to request this and to understand that this is not designed to stimulate a reconciliation.

Requesting Mediation

It is useful if the noninitiator asks the initiator to accept mediation as the vehicle for resolving the issues. In most cases, this request comes as a relief to the initiator, because it promises a faster and less costly resolution of the issues. The request for mediation can be made even if the noninitiator is not yet ready to negotiate a settlement. It may be quite helpful to have an initial meeting with the mediator just to help establish the ground rules for how things will be managed in the household during the time that the noninitiator is getting ready. Because trust may be low and role expectations very confused, this initial consultation can stabilize things and help avoid unintended consequences.

MANAGING GUILT AND BLAME IN AN AFFAIR

In my experience as a mediator, I have found that managing strong feelings of blame, guilt, and humiliation is a challenge of divorce under all circumstances. But when the divorce has been precipitated by the affair of a partner, emotions can be particularly hot. Consider the case of Judy and Rod.

Case Study: Judy and Rod

Judy and Rod have been struggling with their marriage for a long time. They have tried counseling and on numerous occasions have promised each other to try harder in the marriage. Nevertheless, the relationship has slowly continued to deteriorate, and each has begun to feel despair. Rod has begun to work late to delay the frequently unpleasant homecoming, and Judy has begun to grow suspicious. Recently she has become vigilant and has begun to go through his things to check up on him. One day she discovers a credit card receipt for dinner at a fancy restaurant. She knows that she wasn't there with him and confronts him with the receipt. Rod tells her that it was a business meal with a potential client, the chief technology officer for a company in town who might be interested in the software that Rod's company sells. "Who was the person?" Judy demands. "Her name," reports Rod, "is Beverly Thomas." How old is she? What does she look like? Is she single? "I don't know," says Rod, getting defensive. "She is just a potential client."

Judy lets the issue drop for now, but her suspicions are aroused. Two weeks later Rod leaves for a 3-day software convention in Las Vegas. When Judy asks if Beverly will be there, Rod says he doesn't know. So, a day later Judy calls the hotel where the convention is held, poses as an attendee, and asks if Beverly Thomas has checked in yet. The answer is yes. Alarmed, Judy investigates further and discovers that Beverly is registered in room 244. She also finds out that Rod is registered in room 242. It couldn't be a coincidence–that lying bastard is having an affair.

Although not particularly surprised, Judy is furious that Rod had lied and that he probably had been having the affair for a long time, even while they were in marriage counseling. Clearly, the marriage is over, but she is determined that he won't get away with this lying. The divorce will be on her terms, not his. In short order she gets the names of several prominent divorce lawyers and makes appointments to see them.

COMMENTARY: So far, this is not a remarkable story. It occurs in one form or another every day. Assume that Judy is your client and she has her weekly appointment with you the morning before she is to see her first lawyer. What do you do? What do you say? You will, of course, listen to her, acknowledge her intense feelings, and offer sympathy and support. But how will you advise her? Will you suggest any course of action? Will you counsel calm and patience? Or will you duck?

In addition to support and sympathy Judy needs some clear advice. Her best course of action right now is to do nothing. She does not yet need to talk to a lawyer, although that will come in due time. She does not need to teach Rod a lesson or to avenge herself for his perfidy. Judy needs to stay in control of her feelings so that she can begin to think about where she is. She has a choice: she can act on her feelings at the expense of her long-term interests or can avoid acting out while she figures out how to organize her interests. Each therapist will use the tools of his or her training and clinical experience to accomplish this end, but the goal is for Judy to understand the situation and make some clear decisions unclouded by rage and recrimination. Is this marriage truly dead? Although it probably is and has been for some time, she needs to discuss it with her husband, probably with the help of a counselor. She needs Rod to tell her whether he regards the marriage as over and, if not, how he explains what appears to be an extra-marital affair. The decision to end the marriage and the mutual acknowledgment that the marriage is over are the first order of business.

The second thing Judy needs to do is to acknowledge that she must choose between acting on her feelings and acting in her interest. Most of the advice she will get from others and most of her own inclination will push her in the wrong direction. When we feel struck, we want to strike back. When humiliated, we wish to humiliate in return. And when we feel attacked, all our instincts say defend and counterattack. She needs to avoid reflexively striking out at Rod and needs to avoid dramatic confrontations. Assuming that Rod's affair is a signal that the marriage is over, Judy needs to absorb the news and have an opportunity to talk without precipitating a war. This is an important contribution by the therapist, who must convey the following message repeatedly:

> "You have a choice. You can stay in control of your emotions and your future. You do not have to have a struggle, and if you choose correctly, you will be all right when the divorce process is over."

Specifically, Judy needs help to not engage in a blaming contest with Rod, because that will distract her from the real task at hand, which is to build a new life, using her fair share of the family's resources. It is her therapist who can keep her grounded in the realities and help her not slip into a mindless struggle about who is at fault.

AFFAIRS: A CLOSER LOOK

Helping divorcing clients manage the issues surrounding their own affairs or the affairs of their spouses can be challenging. Although there seems to be consensus that in marital therapy affairs should be disclosed, confronted, and perhaps forgiven, there is no such consensus about how to handle the affair in a divorce. When clients manage this issue unwisely, the impact on the divorce can be very destructive.

When a client learns that his or her spouse has been involved with a new lover, the intense feelings of betrayal and humiliation can so destroy the ability to trust that decent divorce becomes unlikely.

> "If I couldn't trust you with other women, how can I trust anything you say about money?"

The feelings are complicated when the affair turns out to be of long standing. The cuckolded spouse wonders whether the other has been lying not only about the affair but about everything else as well. I recall a case in which the wife had caught the husband in an affair 8 years before the divorce and had confronted him. The husband had been contrite and had promised never to see the other woman again. The couple had gone to marriage counseling to work on their relationship and had, seemingly, transcended the affair and continued the marriage. Now, 8 years later, the wife has discovered that the husband lied and had continued his relationship with the other woman. Not only had he continued to maintain the other relationship, but it turned out that he had been paying his lover's rent, bought her a convertible the same year he explained to his wife that they could not afford a new car for her, and, worst of all, paid for her breast enlargement operation. Although this guy sets a record, in my experience, the acute rage and disbelief of his wife when all this came out was almost total.

Most affairs are not as flagrant as this example. A person is lonely because her marriage has grown stale or sour, is tempted by opportunity and enters into a relationship with someone new. Frequently it is a coworker she has known for some time and who has lent a sympathetic ear, slowly becoming a comforting companion. He understands the work that she does and is a friend. The relationship blossoms from a friendship to something more almost on its own steam, so that before she knows it they are in bed together. In many cases, there have been business trips that threw them together in close proximity. And faced with the stress of a declining marriage, the affair feels so good. There are very few marriages, even good ones, that can stand up to an affair. It's like comparing yesterday's black coffee to today's frothy cappuccino.

Do affairs destroy good marriages, or are they only a reflection of marriages already gone sour? I have certainly seen otherwise viable marriages that could have continued at least for a while ended by affairs. In certain situations, a marriage can continue with intense counseling after an affair has been revealed. But I suspect that the majority of affairs develop after the marriage has already deteriorated significantly. I have seen a few but not many cases in which otherwise happily married and emotionally satisfied people get involved in affairs. In most affairs that I have been aware of, the affair is a symptom of something seriously wrong with the marriage.

So, it is not unusual for people to have affairs as marriages unravel, and it is not surprising that the initiator of the divorce will have begun to connect to other people as she accepts that her marriage is over. Having an affair is a way of reassuring herself that she is still attractive and that she will be able to rebuild a social and emotional life after the marriage. So, that which would have been unthinkable during the marriage becomes more acceptable as one spouse departs. But it's not acceptable to the partner. Now, to the strong emotions that accompany any breakup is added the indignation and rage of feeling betrayed. Innumerable novels and movies have been based on this theme, and it continues to have dramatic impact in fiction and in the tabloid press. For a man to be publicly cuckolded is a source of deep humiliation that in some societies can serve as a successful defense to killing one's spouse in retribution. For a woman to be betrayed by a wandering and lecherous husband makes her an object of sympathy and him an object of scorn. So, there is no understating the emotional impact of an affair revealed.

THE IMPACT OF AFFAIRS ON THE DIVORCE

The greatest danger about the revelation of an affair is that it makes it so much easier for the aggrieved spouse to make the affair the central explanation of the divorce. Consider the case of Pam and Gary.

Case Study: Pam and Gary

Pam and Gary had been struggling with their marriage for years. They fought over money. They fought about disciplining the kids. They fought because Gary did not feel that Pam was an adequate housekeeper. And they fought because Gary felt that Pam talked to him in a disrespectful way. Yet, no matter how often he pleaded with her to change, she angrily rejected his requests. Over a period if 5 years, they each engaged in mutual stonewalling, and each grew more distant from the other. Sex diminished and then stopped altogether. Pam gained 30 pounds, and Gary did not find her sexually exciting. When he told her that her weight was a problem for him, she was hurt and angry but did nothing to solve the problem. As the two withdrew from each other, each spent more time in pursuits that didn't involve the other. In time, Gary moved to a separate bedroom. At times each wondered whether he or she ought to consider divorce but did nothing to move in that direction because it was too scary.

Then Gary changed jobs and took a new position working as an account manager for a bank. His new employer used a team approach, and Gary was teamed with Sally, an attractive single woman with whom he quickly established a good rapport. Gary and Sally were a successful team from the beginning and soon were winning praise for their effective recruitment of new business. Working with Sally was fun for Gary, and he enjoyed going into the office in the morning, because he looked forward to spending the day with Sally. Their skills were complementary, and Sally was generous with her praise of her colleague. They were frequently together, having lunch with clients, and often found themselves together in the evening when both stayed late to work on a new account.

Gary and Sally started to become emotionally close and began to share the details of their lives. He told Sally about his frustrations at home, and Sally told him the details of her divorce a year before. A friendship slowly developed over 6 months. Gradually, Gary found himself fantasizing about sex with Sally and felt that she was interested in him. One night, after winning a big account, they went out for dinner to celebrate. As the evening drew to a close, Gary kissed Sally for the first time and found her warm and responsive. Within a few weeks they had slept together, and the affair was on.

Two weeks later, Pam heard a rumor through a friend whose friend worked at the same office as Gary that there was something going on between Gary and a woman at his office. Alarmed, Pam called a lawyer she knew to get the name of a private detective, whom she subsequently hired to follow Gary. Within a week the detective provided Pam with all the evidence she needed, and she confronted Gary that very night. Surprised and feeling ambushed, Gary acknowledged that he had met someone with whom he enjoyed spending time. Pam was furious and told him she wanted him out. He moved out 2 days later, and Pam immediately filed for divorce on grounds of adultery. Pam told her friends that Gary had left her for another woman, and that was the story she told throughout the divorce.

COMMENTARY: As noted, it is seldom that a perfectly good marriage succumbs to an affair. The story of Gary and Pam is the typical case. When a marriage goes sour, it is usually a joint venture of husband and wife, and upon a little investigation we would usually find that each partner contributed to the demise of the marriage. The temptation of the noninitiator is to take refuge in a dramatic story that puts all the blame on the other. Then, he or she is also able to justify in her mind that it is the guilty party who should absorb a disproportionate share of the adverse consequences of the divorce. "You were bad, you suffer" is the posture taken. The difficulty with the affair is that it becomes the story that liberates the "victim" from any responsibility and thus makes it much more difficult to negotiate a reasonable settlement.

In the divorce that followed, Pam never deviated from her position as the aggrieved victim of Gary's infidelity. "You did this to us, so don't expect me to make this easy on you" was her position throughout the prolonged divorce. She punished Gary as much as she could by telling the children that the divorce was caused by his affair, and before long their teenage daughter refused to see Gary because she was so angry at him. Pam refused to do any of the things she could have done to ease the transition for the family. She refused to consider getting a job and refused to consider selling the house that they couldn't afford. Although the case was settled the day before the trial was scheduled, the outcome was bitter. It was years before Gary was able to have a relationship with his daughter. When Gary eventually married Sally, the daughter refused to attend the wedding and exhibited nothing but hostility toward Sally. Pam finally got a job but had lost 3 more years of a career. And Pam and Gary never were able to have a cooperative relationship involving the children.

COMMENTARY: Pam was able to use the affair to relinquish responsibility for her role in the failure of the marriage. That was ultimately to her detriment, and it guaranteed the family a bad divorce. Therapeutic intervention at the beginning of the divorce could have averted this unfortunate outcome. Let us examine two scenarios: one in which Gary is the client and the other in which Pam is the client.

WHAT SHOULD YOUR CLIENT DO IF HE OR SHE HAS HAD AN AFFAIR?

There are several important questions to be answered when your client has had or is having an affair. What does he do? Does he tell or conceal? If his wife finds out, how does he manage it so it doesn't produce an ugly divorce?

I submit that it is not necessary that the client reveal to the spouse that he or she is having an affair. It's kind of late in the game to obsess about honesty and integrity. If the client has been discreet and the affair is not public knowledge and the spouse is unaware of it, nothing is accomplished by telling now. It will focus the spouse exclusively on the affair, justify the assumption of a victim's posture, and generally confuse the divorce. Further, if the client hopes to marry the new love interest someday, identifying him or her now as a "home wrecker" assures that the children will be programmed to resent that person. I understand that many therapists are uncomfortable generally with deceit and secrets and may regard honesty as an important therapeutic goal. I also am aware that couples counselors are extremely uncomfortable with powerful secrets known to the counselor but not to the other spouse. However, the only question now is whether honesty and disclosure serve the objectives of a successful divorce. The requirements of a successful divorce are not the same as those of a successful marriage. If you would encourage your client to disclose as part of marriage therapy, it does not necessarily follow that you also should encourage disclosure as part of a successful divorce.

If the spouse already knows, it is another matter. Now your client's attention must be on damage control, lest the affair become the central legend of the divorce. The aggrieved spouse will be angry and extremely upset. Not only is he or she feeling hurt, rejected, and frightened, but also feels powerful emotions of humiliation and betrayal. Your client needs to be coached to spend a lot of time listening without trying to defend. Initially at least, defending is the last thing he or she should do. Apologies and expressions of contrition help. It is only after the spouse has had an opportunity to tell how he or she feels that he or she will be ready for any discussion that acknowledges that the marriage was dying before the affair. If your client is lucky and listens long enough, the spouse may be ready to hear the message and to join in seeking a constructive divorce. It is counterproductive when your client assumes a belligerent posture. Nothing could be more foolish than to tell the spouse that his or her own behavior is what caused the affair. Although your client will say that the divorce would have happened anyhow, some posture of contrition is necessary to obtain the cooperation of the other spouse. At some level of consciousness, both have some knowledge that both contributed to the divorce. But that will never emerge if they slide into a cycle of attack, defense, and counterattack.

WHEN YOUR CLIENT'S SPOUSE IS HAVING AN AFFAIR

If your client's spouse is having an affair, your task is to help the client understand the affair without using it as an excuse to duck responsibility for the divorce. He or she will need to express the strong feelings of betrayal and rejection and receive empathy and support, but the client also needs help to honestly assess whether the marriage had deteriorated for reasons unconnected to the affair. The affair needs to be placed in perspective so that it is not portrayed as the sole explanation for the divorce. Impulses to punish the other spouse have to be managed, lest they lead to a cycle of mutual recrimination and blame. People can salvage a decent divorce for themselves even when the other spouse has had an affair. The sooner the attention shifts from the recriminations about past behavior to planning for a future life, the sooner your client will heal from the divorce and start a new life. Consider the case of Steve and Jane.

Case Study: Steve and Jane

Steve and Jane had been married for 15 years when Jane told Steve that she wanted a divorce. He was stunned. Although they had had some problems over the years and had had sex only twice during the past 6 months, Steve had always believed that he and Jane would work it out. They had two children, ages 6 and 8, and did many things as a family. Steve was surprised, even blindsided, by Jane's announcement. Through several long evenings, he tried everything he could to talk her out of divorce. He pleaded for the benefit of the children. He pleaded that all they needed was some more time to weather this crisis. He urged Jane to return to counseling with him. But Jane was resolute.

She told him that she simply didn't love him anymore and felt that the life had drained from their relationship years ago. She said that she had agonized about this for years and had struggled unsuccessfully with her growing sense of isolation and loneliness. For years she had pleaded with Steve to talk to her, to share his feelings with her, and not to exclude her from what was happening inside him. But she regarded Steve as closed and guarded. She needed intimacy and close connection and had come to believe that she would never get it from Steve. Approaching age 40, she was determined to have one more chance of closeness with someone before she was too old. Although she didn't believe it would do any good, she agreed to a short round of counseling with Steve in the hope that he would better understand her decision.

So, they went to counseling every week for a month. Here Steve argued for a continuation of the marriage, but Jane held her position and insisted that the marriage was over. As Steve became more frustrated, he also became angry. He started to realize that Jane was proposing to dismantle the life he had struggled to build. In passing comments she had tried to assure him that she wanted him to see the kids as much as he wanted to. And as she spoke, it dawned upon him that she expected him to move out and leave her and the kids in the house. Now he *really* became angry. Then Jane dropped a bomb. During the last session, when Steve was again pleading for another chance, Jane told him that she had started to develop a relationship with a man she had met at work and that she really wanted to be able to pursue that relationship, because she had gone so long without warm companionship.

Now, Steve was beside himself with anger and betrayal. He felt that Jane had suckered him into counseling, knowing that he was hoping to fix the marriage even though she had already decided on divorce. In *his* mind, the divorce had nothing to do with their relationship. Jane was just using their marital difficulties as a pretext to leave the marriage for another man. He hadn't done anything wrong in the marriage. But Jane had betrayed her marital vows and had engaged in adultery. He was the wronged party, and he vowed that she would pay for her behavior. He asked around at work for the name of the most aggressive lawyer he could find. The next week, he filed for divorce, seeking custody of the children and seeking to deny Jane any alimony or marital property. The divorce was a 3-year-long mess with legal fees well into six figures. He didn't get custody. Because the relationship had become so poisonous, visitation with the kids was difficult and awkward. The judge awarded Jane alimony, because she needed it, and awarded her half the marital property. Steve remained bitter and disillusioned, not to mention hundreds of thousands of dollars poorer. He vowed never to marry again.

COMMENTARY: The advice for clients whose spouses are having affairs is consistent with that for the client who is having the affair. When he or she finds out that the spouse has been having an affair, he has the right to grieve and to feel angry. But the same principles still apply about choosing between acting out feelings and acting in one's long-term interests. The clients owe their children the most peaceful divorce they can manage. And in most states the fantasy of punishing the spouse for infidelity will run aground eventually, because few judges are willing and few states permit marital fault to be expressed in the economic resolution of the divorce. There are a few conservative states, mostly southern states like North

Carolina, in which adultery by a wife is a complete bar to alimony and in which the adulterer's paramour can be sued for alienation of affection. But in most states it's not going to matter in the long run, and angry litigation will only leave both spouses poisoned by the years of struggle. Even if they live in a state that permits the adulterous spouse to be punished economically, it is still not worth it, because the entire family will have to live with a legacy of perpetual bitterness.

SUMMARY: THE ROLE OF THE THERAPIST

Your role goes beyond offering sympathy, empathy, and support for a client's feelings, although these are an integral part of therapy. You must function as the client's chief reality tester. An equally important component of therapy is to promote the client's ability to take responsibility in the divorce. This critical step cannot wait long for insight by the client. It must be advanced as the initial agenda.

> "Yes, you feel betrayed. You feel angry and scared and humiliated. And you have a right to feel those things, and it's appropriate that you feel those things. We will address them together in therapy over time. But there are immediate decisions to be made. Now, what are you going to *do*?"

At this point, the client is undoubtedly getting numerous messages from lawyers, friends, and other would-be advisors who encourage fighting, blaming, and anything but taking responsibility and insisting on fairness. But what such advice invariably lacks is a vision that would create a logical link between a successful divorce in the future and a sense of restraint in the present.

In a divorce, the therapist is the one who pushes the client to act responsibly in his or her own interest. It is your role to help the client balance past and future visions and to emphasize that good marriages do not fail suddenly. The development of a failed marriage—even when there is an affair—takes years. Marriages tend to die from a thousand cuts rather than one sudden mortal blow. The client needs help in constructing a realistic history of the divorce so that the behavior of both spouses is appropriately understood and a constructive vision of the future can be pursued.

BUILDING THE VISION OF THE FUTURE

When we train divorce mediators, we teach that a major strategic goal is to shift the client's focus from the past to the future. This is one of the significant differences between mediation and conventional adversarial divorce. The latter is replete with doctrines that rivet the attention of the spouses on the past. Who contributed more? Who is more worthy? Who has been the more important parent? Whose behavior caused the divorce? What is the standard to which she has become entitled? All of these questions usually reflect the very disagreements that caused the divorce in the first place, and the spouses are utterly unable to reconcile their clashing view of history. The "dialogue" drives the parties further apart and deepens the distrust and mutual alienation. Nevertheless, lawyers continue to fan these flames, because they think it will improve their negotiating position and because they think these arguments might sway the judge in the remote eventuality that the case goes to trial.

I often tell clients that, although I have mediated thousands of divorces I have never once succeeded in getting two spouses to agree on a common history of their relationship. Accordingly, I regard the likelihood of doing that with this particular couple as nil and will not support the attempt. As a mediator, I have very little interest in helping people to vindicate history.

So, if we have so little interest in the past, what do we have? Our role is to help clients in building a viable vision of the future. Whatever contribution we can make is based on a large knowledge base that the client probably does not have. We know that the majority of people remarry within 5 years. We know that most people will rebuild their social lives and that most children will settle down and do well. We know that, if both spouses thrive, the children will also thrive. And we know that, when the parents retain the ability to cooperate around issues related to the children, the children adapt well to the divorce. We also know that the chance of a second divorce's occurring is much increased by a bitter first divorce and that the baggage of a bitter ex-spouse and alienated children increases the chances that the new relationship will fail. We know people do better in divorce when the issues are resolved quickly so that they do not have to endure an interminable limbo. We know families do better when they do not exhaust their money on legal fees for protracted legal proceedings. We know divorcing partners do better when they treat each other well and when both feel that the settlement was fair. And all these things we know provide a compelling vision for the client that establishes a standard against which to compare the utility of any proposed plan of action.

With any client I encourage a vision of the future that assumes that:

1. They will probably develop a significant new relationship within a few years.
2. Their ex-spouse will also develop such a relationship.
3. Their children will thrive only if both of them thrive.
4. They need to work on minimizing the emotional and financial cost of the divorce process.
5. They will need to develop an efficient mechanism for dispute resolution.
6. They will need to help their children be comfortable in both households.
7. Their children will need to like and respect the other parent's new significant other.

With this future scenario articulated, we are then in a position to evaluate any proposed action in terms of whether it advances or retards the achievement of this vision. It does not matter whether the end of the marriage has been triggered by an affair. Do I seek mediation or litigation? Do I seek more than half the assets, or do I settle for half? Do I seek an aggressive, litigious lawyer, or do I seek a collaborative lawyer? Do I try to minimize the support I pay, or do I endeavor to make the best use of resources for every family member? Do I file on fault grounds or no-fault grounds? Do I move out of the house sooner or later? Do I withhold visitation in an attempt to get more child support? These and many other strategic and tactical decisions can be analyzed more fruitfully only after the client has developed a vision of the future. The therapist can continually refocus the client, balancing validation of the client's pain and betrayal with the need to pursue a vision of the future that will serve the needs of the entire family.

MANAGING THE CRISIS

Once the decision to divorce has been made and communicated, couples enter into a difficult period in which it is easy to bumble into a bad divorce. All the civility achieved when the first stage is handled well can be squandered during the ensuing months if the crises that follow are not handled correctly. The challenge, of course, is to manage the tumultuous emotions swirling through the house. Although some couples separate as soon as the divorce is announced, most couples will continue to live in the same house while they decide how to manage the separation.

But living in the same house after the decision to divorce is very difficult—for numerous reasons that we will discuss in the next chapter. Hostility is almost inevitable. Because there are no established protocols and because communication is difficult, there are many opportunities to accidentally step on each other's toes. Unrealized expectations, insensitive remarks, screw-ups about who was supposed to pick up the children, and other missteps and misunderstandings are inevitable. These difficulties naturally affect divorcing couples, even those who are not living in the same house, as new routines are developed and new modes of communication are established. A wide variety of problems and glitches can arise, and therein lies the problem.

When people are on good terms, they do not normally impute negative intentions to each other's actions. When my friend steps on my toe, I automatically assume that it was accidental and unintentional. I say "Ouch!", he apologizes, and it is forgotten. But when someone who is not my friend and may even be my adversary steps on my toe, I'm not so sure it was accidental. Maybe he was being malicious and trying to inflict pain. The event is the same, but the intention imputed to him by me may radically differ. And if I conclude that he was trying to hurt me, I become really angry. Not only will I be wary of him in the future and ensure he doesn't get within striking distance of my toes, but I just might retaliate to show him that I'm no wimp and that I can push back. Now, suppose that it really *was* an accident, but I decide it was intentional. My retaliation strikes him as a hostile act, and he reacts with distrust and further retaliation. Within a short time we are at war. This is what I call a "death spiral."

The vicious cycle of attack and counterattack is the death spiral of relationships that can easily occur early in the divorce. It is inevitable that each partner steps on the toes of the other, at least figuratively. As each begins to infer hostile intent, each begins to retaliate, and the atmosphere soon becomes poisonous. The situation rapidly deteriorates into a pattern of mutual "negative attribution." Each one starts to assume the worst about the intentions of the other. Negative attribution leads to actions that both incorrectly perceive as necessary for self-protection. So, the husband, worried that his wife will run up a large credit card bill, cancels her credit card without telling her. She is humiliated when she goes to the store and has her card declined. She is also frightened that he is going to use his superior financial position to bully her in the divorce. So, she seeks rescue from a lawyer who immediately files the divorce papers and asks the court to freeze the husband's assets. As the couple proceeds to ever more hostile feelings, each party comes to believe that it is the other one who is engaged in dirty tactics, and this belief justifies retaliation in kind. It does not occur to either that the other is simply frightened and acting out of ignorance. The lawyers serve as agents to intensify this process rather than stepping in to impose calm and to educate the couple so that they are less fearful of each other.

Whether your client is the initiator or the noninitiator, both partners should be aware that the other spouse is going to make mistakes. He may run late, she may exceed their credit limit. Events such as these are susceptible to erroneous interpretation, and both parties must be careful about how they communicate with each other. It is understandable that both are touchy and reactive, but they must make a concerted effort to steer away from confrontations, maintain a civil and respectful tone, and exercise the consideration expected of any adult roommate. They also need to duck when the other is provocative. If one offends the other, an apology should be readily forthcoming. Lastly, they should be counseled against listening to the Greek chorus of interested bystanders who encourages them to seek legal "protection" against each other's perceived attacks–as well as against lawyers who step in to offer such "protection." My experience has taught me that the therapist is one of the few people in the client's life who can help the client control this process and avoid this destructive cycle.

CONCLUSION

The ways in which couples manage the early stages of divorce largely determine how well or poorly the divorce will turn out. Couples that manage their feelings without resorting to acrimonious litigation have the best chance of a cooperative divorce. Couples that lose control are doomed to a bad divorce. Lucky couples will have wise advisors available to help them steer away from the destructive behaviors that follow their instinctive impulses and bad advice from well-meaning but misinformed friends and colleagues. In more cases than not, that advisor can be the therapist who is willing to intervene with emotional support and practical guidance and stay with the client through the process.

4 Managing the Separation

In every divorce there comes a time when the couple must separate. Divorcing couples do not do well when they try to live together for a long time. Rancor increases and the opportunities for hurt feelings and confrontations blossom. Once the decision to divorce has been made, neither partner can really live in peace until the spouses are living in separate dwellings. Trying to share the same home is stressful for many reasons. The couple has no routines or protocols for defining their relations or activities together. Does she do his laundry or cook his meals? Does he continue to deposit his paycheck into the joint account? Do they sleep in separate bedrooms or stay in the same one? Who moves out of the bedroom, if either? Should they sit down to dinner as a family, as they did for many years, or should they have separate meals? Should they try to have conversations with each other, or should they not? In either case, they will feel awkward trying to make polite conversation and will feel equally uncomfortable living in stony silence. What about friends? Do they continue to entertain friends and socialize with other couples—a process uncomfortable for all—or do they just live separate social lives? And what about dating? Living in the same house makes each acutely aware of when the other comes and goes, and thereby jealousy is created and stoked. Because there are no clearly defined roles, the opportunities for mistakes and missed cues abound.

There are myriad practical and emotional issues. The couple may experience role confusion. They are used to turning to each other for advice and solace. In some cases, they may have been estranged for so long that this doesn't apply. But for most couples, at least one of them—particularly the noninitiator—is inclined to seek the help of the other. But when the other is the source of the pain that is so troubling, it doesn't help to seek relief from the spouse. In fact, it makes matters worse. And when one of the partners is still resisting the divorce, the situation is even more uncomfortable, because the noninitiator continues to importune the initiator to change his or her mind or misinterprets any act of kindness or gentleness as a chance for reconciliation. Then, dashed hopes for reconciliation lead to renewed feelings of betrayal and another round of condemnation and bickering.

Living in a house with a dead marriage is bad for the entire family. When involved in a divorce, the therapist should make facilitating the separation a priority. This chapter is designed to familiarize therapists with some of the issues that typically arise during the separation stage and to arm you with facts and practical suggestions to present to your clients.

PSYCHOLOGICAL DYNAMICS OF THE MOVE: INITIATOR VERSUS NONINITIATOR

For the noninitiator, the actual separation is an important event, because it makes the divorce a reality. For some noninitiators, the move triggers an acute sense of crisis. If the initiator is moving out, it triggers an acute sense of abandonment. And if the noninitiator moves out under pressure, he is likely to be very depressed moving into quarters that are typically very spartan as compared to the marital home. The anxiety associated with the anticipation of the move and the immediate aftermath of the move can be severe, and the therapist will do well to have the client anticipate and manage these strong feelings.

WHO SHOULD LEAVE?

It is my experience that in most divorces involving children the husband is the one who moves out. There is a compelling logic to this, because it is still mothers who have primary residential custody most of the time. Even when the parties have joint custody, the mother is most often the primary administrator of the daily affairs of the children. If the parties are in agreement about their respective roles and responsibilities regarding parenting and the father does not fear that he will be deprived of reasonable access, then he is more likely to be the one to move. In some cases the father would like to try a different arrangement but "gives in" because he doesn't see any alternative and can't convince his wife to try something new. An increasing number of fathers struggle to get equal time with the children, and some of them succeed. But even when this happens, chances are good that the mother will continue to stay in the marital home and at least for a while the father moves out.

Although most husbands ultimately move out, many endure a lengthy struggle before they finally do so. There are four reasons this happens.

1. *Fear that such a move will be used to their legal disadvantage later.* Many laypeople believe that, if they move, their spouse will be able to accuse them of "abandonment" and use this accusation to punish them in court. This is untrue. Remember, almost no divorce cases ever go to trial, and in the few that do, judges are aware that once a marriage is over someone has to move. So, the fear of being accused of abandonment and desertion can be easily allayed. The wife is probably desperate for the husband to move. She will almost certainly be willing to write a letter in which she acknowledges that she is asking him to move to benefit the mental health of the family. With such a letter in hand, he is completely protected against subsequent accusations of abandonment.

2. *Fear that, by moving, the husband forfeits his property rights in the house.* This is also completely untrue. If the couple owns the house together, he will continue to maintain his ownership interest after he leaves, and the settlement will eventually have to address how he gets his share of ownership of the marital home. Some men worry that, once they move out, they will not be allowed back in if they change their minds. This may be true, because courts will be reluctant to risk the conflict that may develop if he reoccupies the house after a lengthy period of separate residence. He may be able to reduce this risk by asking his wife to include in her letter a statement that he is entitled to reoccupy the house at any time if he chooses. Although a woman might resist the idea that the husband could move back in, she must weigh the low probability that he will actually want to move back in later against his possible refusal to move out if this is not agreed

3. *Fear that a move will weaken the husband's negotiation position.* Many lawyers tell their clients not to move, because they fear that such a move will compromise their negotiating position. Some men are hoping that their wife will agree to sell the house and move to smaller quarters. Some may fear that the wife will withhold the children or insist on more support than the husband can afford. Because the husband's con-

tinued presence in the house is an irritant to the wife, his lawyer believes that the very discomfort caused to the wife by the continued residence of the husband will provide an incentive to her to make other concessions just to get him out. Many lawyers also worry that, by moving out and leaving the wife in place with the children, the male client will inadvertently establish a "status quo" that will later be continued by a court even if the man cannot afford it.

I cannot say that such a ploy is ineffective, because it may indeed induce concessions from the wife on occasion. But more often it does not work and results in rising tensions and ever increasing bitterness.

4. *Fears about supporting two households.* Many men do not know how they will be able to afford decent housing for themselves while continuing to pay the bills for the existing household. Most middle-class couples live right at or just beyond the financial edge. They have little in the way of reserves and live paycheck to paycheck. So, the cost of another residence looms as an insurmountable financial obstacle, and they fear that moving will plunge them further into debt.

WHEN THE WIFE MOVES OUT

Although it is more common for husbands to move out, there are several scenarios in which the wife moves out first.

1. *The couple has decided that the house will be sold and that the wife will move first to get the kids settled in their new house.* In this scenario, the couple is cooperating, and there is no problem.

2. *The wife is desperate to be separated, and the husband absolutely refuses to move, even when it is clear that the wife will be the primary parent and that it would be more economical for him to move.* In this situation we usually find that the wife was the initiator and that the husband is having trouble dealing with the divorce and the changes that are required. So, the wife is faced with a choice of living together until the husband finally decides to move or of moving herself with the kids in order to force the separation. It is a strong and gutsy woman indeed who refuses to be held hostage to her husband's intransigence. The alternative, to continue living together, requires that she accept a period of limbo that she finds unacceptable. I have seen women use their willingness to move and their preparation to move as a way of convincing the husband that he cannot keep the marriage together by force of will.

A move under these conditions can cause a good deal of economic disorder, because the wife rents a house large enough to accommodate the children and this rent, combined with the costs of the marital home, really stretches the couple's budget. If the mother will continue as the primary residential parent of the children, the move will affect children at a time when stability is preferred. Because the move is not the mother's first choice but is undertaken only out of necessity, it may be characterized by feelings of resentment at the dislocation to which she and the children are subjected. There is much work for the therapist here in helping the couple, or coaching one of the spouses, to see that this turns out to have a sensible conclusion. Here again the therapist can be helpful by continually reminding the client that the move, however painful, is a necessary part of the transition and if done in a timely and graceful manner can help achieve peace of mind for everyone and improve the chances of a good divorce.

3. *The father is the primary parent.* Occasionally, we find a wife moving out because the husband is to be the primary parent. She moves and leaves him at home with the children. Typically, the child or children are older and are adamant about staying in the house. The wife trusts the parenting abilities of the father and wants to pursue her own objectives. As we observed in an earlier case study, a couple in their late 40s with two older teenagers and the wife in law school. The couple decided that the wife, who had been a homemaker for many years, had earned the right to devote herself to her studies and that it was the husband's turn to shoulder the lion's share of parenting responsibilities for a while. Note that the way the couple framed the decision did not attach a stigma to the wife or label her a "bad" or neglectful mother.

There are situations in which, for any number of reasons, fathers emerge as the primary parent. When this is the best way to reorganize the family, mothers need help in creating a public definition that avoids the stigma of the bad mother. We generally label these as "joint custody" even when the father is, in fact, primary. It makes it much easier for the mother to let go without fearing being condemned as a bad mother. Clearly, the therapist can be most helpful in creating this "frame" for the couple.

GUIDING CLIENTS THROUGH THE MOVE

The therapist involved in a divorce is in a unique position to help the client understand the costs and benefits of moving. It is the therapist rather than the lawyer who is able to speak with authority about the psychological impact of staying together and the psychological benefits of moving out. This may indeed be a situation in which the therapist and the lawyer give contradictory advice. Lawyers won't like it and may even communicate their displeasure. Stand your ground. This is your area of expertise and your turf.

Generally, a move should occur as soon as practical after the decision to divorce is made. It is at this point that there is still residual goodwill between the parties, notwithstanding a lot of anger and other strong feelings. It is at this point that the clients have to be directed to begin focusing on achieving a good divorce. And an essential feature of a good divorce is the retention of the very goodwill that will be lost by living in a state of deadlock and limbo for a long time. Similarly, every increase in bitterness and a sense of bad will increases the probability that this hostility will be carried over into new lives and sabotage them. If it is clear that one will have to leave eventually, the refusal to leave just reduces the residual trust between the partners and delays any healing that needs to begin. As a therapist, you are uniquely situated to be the guide for this perilous passage of your clients.

HELPING CLIENTS TO SOLVE THE PROBLEMS OF MOVING OUT

Negotiating and executing a decent separation is one of the last important tasks of the marriage. Although it may strike one as ironic, the spouses have a strong mutual interest in achieving a rapid and cooperative separation. For the most part, the things they worry about–kids and money–have to be resolved cooperatively. Here is where the therapist can coach either one or both parties effectively. The therapist may do this on his or her own or in support of a mediator. Once again, the therapist is in a teaching role. As this is the beginning of the couple's negotiation, the therapist must teach the client appropriate language for recruiting the spouse's cooperation rather than evoking resistance. We will discuss negotiation in greater detail in Chapter 8 when we look at negotiation of the settlement. But because negotiation skills are crucial in determining who moves out, some highlights are presented here.

It is important to note that many issues of the divorce will not be solved before the separation. For example, many men fear that they will lose access to their children or be unable to support two households. Negotiating issues surrounding the separation does not mean having all the answers. Instead, it means creating a cooperative environment and inviting the spouse to engage in joint problem solving.

> "I think it would be a good idea for me to move, and I know that you think so too. But I am worried about two things, and I need your help to solve the problems. As soon as we begin to get a grip on these I will move. First, I am worried about how I will get enough time with the children if I move out, and I need some reassurance from you about that. Second, I do not know where the money will come from to pay for this, and I need your help to figure out how we will pay for both households."

Note two elements that categorize the statements above, because we will be returning to them frequently.

Neutral Language

There is no accusation, and there is no hostility. Compare this to the following statement:

> "If you want me to move, then you better quit spending so much money and go out and get a job and stop expecting me to do everything for you."

This points an accusatory finger at the spouse and will elicit an angry and defensive response. Neutral language focuses on "I" statements rather than "you" statements and never includes blame or accusation. "I need to move out for all our sakes" is a neutral statement, as is "I don't know how we can afford the second household."

Problem Solving as a Joint Endeavor

The client must learn not to begin with a position about how to solve the problem, for many men this is an especially important lesson because they tend to be oriented to problem solving and often fail to understand that women may process difficult problems differently from them. Women going through divorce, in the cases I have worked on, have usually needed to wrestle with the emotional implications longer than the men have, and they have needed men to be patient while they do it. "Can you help me solve it?" is an invitation to cooperate that is difficult to resist.

> "I am concerned that the children get to spend enough time with me to maintain our relationship, and I want to do my fair share of parenting so that we can both get on with our lives. What are your thoughts on how we manage this?"

Contrast this to:

> "I've decided that the only fair way to work out our parenting is to have an even 50/50 split of time with the children."

The wife is not yet ready for problem solving, and this ready-made solution can only elicit anger and resentment.

Statements should also be free of implicit or explicit threats that are designed to foist a preconceived solution on an unwilling partner. One does not begin with a position such as:

> "I insist that I get equal time with the kids. I won't settle for anything less than 50/50, and I'm not going anywhere until you agree to my proposed schedule!"

Positions such as these are bound to induce resistance and need to be avoided. The same sentiment can be expressed in neutral language.

> "I know we need to separate and I want to move out as soon as we can solve this."

Although both say essentially the same thing, the latter evokes resistance, while the former does not. This is not just semantics. It is the key to keeping the discussion constructive.

As we will see in the next chapter, negotiation does not follow a predetermined script, and even the most neutral statements can be met with hostility and suspicion. However, suspicion and anger can also be met with effective neutral language.

> "I understand that you are angry and scared, but I also believe that we will never fully agree on history. Why don't we see if we can come to agreement on the future?"

This is a far more productive way to create an atmosphere of negotiation than

> "This divorce is as much your fault than mine and if you had been more affectionate you might have received what you wanted from me!"

Counterattack inevitably begets another round of attack. Coach your clients to not attack and, when attacked, not to defend. It is the best way to arrest the slow slide into a war of attrition.

Separation involves problems related to money, children, and lifestyle. These problems will be not resolved easily or without struggle. Both partners are frightened. It is all too easy to slip into blame and recrimination for the divorce as a way to justify why the other spouse is responsible for the trouble and therefore should bear the burden of solution. The critical task at this stage is to maintain a tone of cooperation instead of confrontation and to create an interim arrangement that will remain in place during the separation until the negotiation of more permanent arrangements.

WHERE TO MOVE?

Once the decision is made that one of the spouses will move, the couple needs to discuss where that spouse will move.

Many men's initial impulse is to move closer to where they work to reduce their commuting time. Other men are eager to move to a more urban area because the social opportunities for single people are better. Both of these are legitimate reasons for choosing where to live. But if they have children and hope to have their children spend much time with them, they must consider what factors facilitate their children's willingness to come and spend time with them.

Case Study: Bob and Patty

Bob and Patty separated 5 months ago. Patty and the children continued to reside in the marital home located in a New Jersey suburb of Manhattan. Bob wanted to reduce his commute, which took over an hour each way. He had moved to Hoboken, a small city just across the Hudson River from Manhattan. Bob had succeeded in reducing his commute to 20 minutes each way and had found an apartment in a complex right in the center of the social action. He was very pleased with the move. But Bob's children were not so pleased. Tina, age 12, and James, age 9, complained whenever they had to go to their father's for the weekend. Bob and Patty, like most couples, had agreed to alternate weekends with the children, and Bob had also committed to spending Wednesday evenings with the children. Because it was impractical to drive the kids 40 minutes each way on a weekday evening, Bob would drive to Patty's house to take the kids out to dinner. This only worked sometimes. Often one or both children claimed that they had too much homework to go out to dinner. They wanted Bob to spend the evening in the house with them so that he could visit and help with homework at the same time. Bob had tried this numerous times but felt increasingly uncomfortable being in what had become Patty's house. And Patty, who had been eager to see Bob move out, did not welcome the invasion of her privacy. So, Wednesday evenings were not particularly satisfactory to anyone.

Weekends were not much fun either. James was a dedicated athlete at 9 years of age. He played soccer in the fall and baseball in the spring. He had practice almost every afternoon and games almost every weekend. So, when he had a weekend at his dad's place, it meant that he would have to miss a game or that his dad would have to spend the weekend driving back and forth, or he would skip the weekend to stay with his mother. Tina also had her problems with the weekends. She was in junior high school and was a popular child with a large circle of friends. Her friends usually met for parties or a movie at least one evening of the weekend, and Tina resented having to miss the fun to go to her dad's house. Tina also played soccer and sang in the school chorus, both of which required attendance at weekend events. All this put Bob in a difficult position. Either he spent the entire weekend driving back and forth, or he refused and told the children they would have to spend the weekend in Hoboken with him. When this happened he found himself going crazy trying to entertain two sullen and disgruntled kids. Increasingly he found that one or both children would plead to be allowed to skip a weekend, and this created tension with Patty, because she wanted some time to herself and was resentful when she had to give up her weekend off because the children didn't want to go to Bob's place.

COMMENTARY: Bob's dilemma is a common one. But the consequences can be serious because they can ruin the ability of the family to adjust well to the divorce. A successful parenting schedule is one in which children can share their parent's lives without undue disruption of their own. So, it comes down to this. If a father expects to maintain a robust relationship with his children, he needs to live within their social orbit. Once he moves beyond that boundary, problems are likely. The problems will arise with all children but will be particularly acute with teenagers. In adolescence the developmental task of children is to begin to separate from their parents. Their peers become much-preferred companions. Most teens don't particularly want to hang out with their parents, who, they increasingly feel, are just a source of embarrassment. So, when a teenage child spends the weekend with a parent, she may only actually be with the parent for a few hours as she spends most of her waking hours with friends and in activities apart from the parent. But, if the parent interposes himself and insists that she hang out with him, he gets nothing but a grumpy kid. Fathers move away at the expense of an easy relationship with their children. So, as in all strategic divorce decisions, a little intervention from the therapist can avoid a lot of grief.

Although it is usually the husband who moves out, wives do move with the children when the husband digs in his heels and refuses to move. The considerations of proximity discussed above with respect to the husband's move still apply when the woman moves, but some practical considerations may make it more difficult for the mother to stay close to the marital home. Because she must find a home suitable for herself and the children, her practical options may be more limited because she has to look farther afield to find affordable housing. The therapist may be helpful in coaching the wife to carefully explain her dilemma to the husband so that he does not impute destructive motives to the wife when she moves out of the neighborhood. I have had cases in which husbands have changed their minds and moved when they fully understood the choices available to the wife.

THE NEED FOR A REAL HOME

When money is tight and the pressure is on to get separated, it may be tempting for your client, if he (or she) is the one moving out, to find the smallest, least expensive, apartment available. This is a mistake and should be avoided. For both the client's welfare and the welfare of his children, he needs a real home. He's too old to resume the life of an undergraduate. He needs someplace to come home to at the end of the day that is comfortable and aesthetically pleasing. He needs enough space to accommodate the children for overnights and to have a little privacy when they are there. Sleeping bags on the floor may seem like fun at first, but the novelty wears off quickly. Children need their own rooms and, depending on their age and sex, it may not work to ask them to share a bedroom. It is not reasonable to ask a teenage daughter to share a room with her 10-year-old brother and will cause her to resist staying overnight.

Setting up a real home requires some time, energy, and skill. Some men have it, while others are clueless. He will need to shop for furniture to supplement whatever he takes from the marital home. There is plenty of inexpensive but attractive furniture on the market, and he should seek consultation among his friends to find someone who can help. And there is more to setting up a home than just buying furniture. Although it may appear to fall outside the purview of "therapy," the man should be encouraged to furnish his home with amenities that make it comfortable–sheets and towels, bedding and pillows, and placemats for the table. Equipping a kitchen requires pots, utensils, dishes, glassware, flatware, and condiments and spices. A single trip or two to a good department store can be all that is needed to fully equip an apartment, but it has to be planned well. I find that too many men underestimate the importance of setting up a real home and then don't understand why they feel so depressed when they return to their homes at night. Men need to be coached to do this well, and their wives need to be coached about how important it is. It is too easy in the anxiety about making ends meet to assume that the father can get by with minimal housing. But this is a recipe for big trouble later and must be attended to early on.

Some comment is appropriate here on the role wives should play in helping the husband set up his new home. I have seen numerous cases in which wives did this and it worked out all right. Some men may be so helpless that from the wife's perspective he will never move if she doesn't help. On the other hand, I think men should be encouraged to set up their own homes without relying on their wives to take care of them. It is better for the husband to start taking care of himself and seek help, if necessary, from friends or even professional decorators. When the wife begins the husband's move by taking care of him, it often becomes difficult for her to draw a line where to stop. And when she finally says "enough is enough," he may react with resentment and anger.

FINANCIAL IMPLICATIONS

Setting up a proper home requires significant financial outlay precisely when the couple is feeling most strapped. Nevertheless, the need for a real home is more than a simple issue of material comfort–it is also a matter of mental health for the parent and the children. If the two partners have savings, now is the time to spend some of them. Depending on how much furniture the couple already has, furnishing a two-bedroom apartment should be possible for $3,000–8,000. Setting up a kitchen costs between $2,500 and $3,000, depending on what is already owned. So, about $10,000 (in round numbers) should do the job well. Additionally, a security deposit will be required that can vary from 1 to 2 months' rent, and, depending on the rental market where they live, they may also have to pay a broker's fee that typically runs about 1 month's rent. To find and rent a two-bedroom apartment, again depending on local markets, can cost from $2,500 to $7,500. So, while vast sums are not needed to set up a real home, $10,000–15,000 is a realistic range and requires the couple to do some planning to make it happen.

WHO PAYS?

Some couples faced with the need to create a new residence get into conflicts over how the cost of the move will be distributed between them. Typically, the wife wants the husband to absorb the cost from his share of the marital assets, and he wants her to share in at least part of the transition costs of the move. More often than not, the move will occur before the financial settlement has been worked out, and we don't want the move to aggravate insecurities about the settlement.

I generally suggest that the portion of the expenses that are strictly transition costs should be shared. The broker's fee and the cost of moving are transition costs. But the expenses that are incurred to acquire items that will belong to one of the partners should be paid for out of that partner's assets. The security deposit is property belonging to the renter. Furniture and equipment is personally owned property. These should be paid from that person's share of the marital assets.

DIVIDING THE HOUSEHOLD GOODS

Although it may seem unimportant in the large scheme of things, the division of household property can trigger struggles and resentments between the separating partners. He is leaving and needs to set up a household. Although he may be reluctant to disturb the existing household, he also feels that it is unfair to require him to spend his money on furniture while she keeps everything. She protests that the household shouldn't be "torn up" and that he should make do.

One solution is for the remaining spouse to purchase the departing spouse's interest in the furnishings. Although this may seem logical, it often falls apart over issues of valuation. The couch that they bought 3 years ago for $2,000 is now worth $500 at a house sale. Moreover, when he goes to buy a similar couch, it will cost him $2,000. So, is he to be compensated with one-half of replacement cost ($1,000) or one-half of current cost ($250)? I have seen many bitter fights over this issue. It is very difficult to agree on a fair price for buying out the furnishings.

Unless couples can easily and spontaneously divide the furnishings, I suggest the following. They make a list of all the household goods. They toss a coin, and the coin toss winner gets first pick. Then the other picks and so on until there are two lists. Each will have to replace some things and each will lose a few things he or she would have preferred to have. But the system is fair and avoids ongoing resentment. I believe that children are able to manage with various pieces of furniture coming and going; so, the notion of maintaining continuity for the sake of the children must be tempered by the need to maintain a sense of mutual fairness between the parents.

An exception to this method applies to family heirlooms and gifts. If the wife's mother gave them Grandmother's dining room set, it should go to the wife. And if the husband's parents gave them a valuable antique, it should go to the husband. Although there are legal claims that a spouse can make if the parents made a gift to the couple, the emotional costs of making that claim are not worth the cost, and the item should go back to the family from whence it came.

The important goal is to achieve a move quickly and amicably into a dwelling that serves the needs of the family. Disagreements over the relatively small amounts of capital involved should not be permitted to create a deadlock. Although I generally discourage credit card spending, this is one of the few times that I would suggest use of debt, if necessary, to facilitate the move. If the couple needs a small home equity loan to finance the move, they should take it. The debt will be managed as part of the overall settlement. So long as they stay within reasonable cost parameters, the additional debt will not cause a problem.

A HOUSING STRATEGY TO AVOID

Before leaving this chapter, I want to address an idea that often appeals to couples whose primary concern is avoiding change for their children. At some point in the early discussions, one partner proposes that the children stay in the house and the parents alternate living in the house with the kids. For example, one couple I saw recently proposed that the parents would each occupy the house every other week while the children stayed in the house. There are many reasons that this concept, often called "birdnesting," is a bad idea. First, it is expensive. It requires three dwellings instead of two, as each parent needs his or her own apartment in addition to the house. If they get one apartment and share it as well as the house they are now sharing two dwellings and in effect never really separate. The second problem is that this arrangement keeps them tied financially. They have to continually coordinate expenses in the house, and if they also share an apartment, they also have to coordinate expenses for that. As a consequence, they have no privacy with respect to each other.

But the most important reason not to do this is that it will inevitably fall apart in a short time. As each starts to build a new social life, the strains of this arrangement will begin to show. No new girlfriend or boyfriend will tolerate sleeping in the same bed vacated just yesterday by the ex-spouse. And no new significant other will tolerate for long moving between two residences. It also falls apart because the complications for the parents of moving between two residences and constantly coordinating with their ex-spouses are just too great. The arrangement prevents either from really settling into a new home and starting a new life. I have never seen this work for more than a few months. The arrangement also reflects confusion about the organization of the needs of parents and adults. The desire to protect children from change and the willingness of the parents to accept any price that results from that posture is illusory at best. If they wear themselves out trying to protect children from the reality of the divorce, they won't be of much use to the kids. Everyone in the family must accept a degree of change in order for the family to adapt well. To subordinate all of the parent's needs to those of the kids means that nobody will thrive over time. The needs of all family members are equally important.

THE ROLE OF THE THERAPIST

The actual physical separation of the couple is a task of major importance and is fraught with myriad potential difficulties. This is a topic in which the therapist can make a great difference for the client, whether the therapist is coaching the couple or just one individual. Therapists should not be timid about weighing in with opinions about how to do this well. Clients need help in understanding how their fears about separation can interfere with the practical tasks to be accomplished. They also need to be reminded of what they are trying to accomplish by way of a cooperative divorce and how the selection and furnishing of the second dwelling can have an important impact.

However, if there is a developing struggle over time with the children, a father is more likely to refuse to go. Even when a man is willing to move, it is common for his lawyers to counsel him not to do so until all issues are resolved. In these cases we can expect his wife to become increasingly angry, because she wants him out of the house; if the situation goes on long enough, the couple become prime candidates for some kind of incident that leads to a domestic violence complaint and the forcible removal of the husband.

5 Law and Divorce

As a therapist, you must be knowledgeable about divorce laws and procedures to provide accurate information for confused clients and, even more importantly, to recognize and dispel common myths about divorce law. This does not mean, of course, that you must be familiar with every nuance and facet of this highly complex and arcane system. That would be beyond your purview as a therapist. General familiarity should be sufficient to provide guidance to clients as they proceed through the divorce process. This chapter will provide you with an overview of divorce laws and procedures. In Chapter 6, I will introduce you to the legal culture where these laws are interpreted and enacted.

WHAT IS DIVORCE, LEGALLY SPEAKING?

The answer to this question starts with another question: What is a marriage? A marriage is a public ceremony sanctioned by the state that creates a new legal status for the two people getting married. Many years ago, it was not legal for people to have sex until they married, making marriage essential to human connection, not to mention procreation. Marriage also gave couples certain rights and obligations with respect to each other. Each acquired the right to inherit part of the other's estate. Each acquired certain economic responsibilities for the other. Each could demand that the other maintain a monogamous relationship. All of these were inherent in the legal status created when they made the state, in effect, a third party to the relationship.

Marriage was intended to be permanent, ending only when "death do you part." So, people who wanted to end the marriage had to offer compelling reasons to the state why the marriage should end and had to obtain the permission of the state. The state was–and remains–the only entity that can dissolve a marriage, because only the state is empowered to create the marriage. Divorce is simply the reversal of the official edict that a couple is married. And since only the state can declare a couple to be divorced, only the state can establish the rules that apply to the dissolution of marriage. The court of each state is the institution that carries out the law of that state. That is why the couple must go to court to get divorced.

There are three sets of legal requirements that must be satisfied before the court will grant a divorce. First, one has to establish that the court has jurisdiction over the marriage. Jurisdiction is based on residence; so, one must establish that he or she has been living in the state long enough to qualify as a legal resident. Once the jurisdiction of the court is established, one must establish grounds for divorce. Grounds are the reason offered to the state why it should dissolve the marriage. Each state legislature has laws stating the reasons the state will accept as a basis of divorce. (We will elaborate on these laws later on.) Having established grounds and jurisdiction, the court must be satisfied that the couple has resolved the issues of divorce: custody of the children, support of the children, support for each spouse, and division of the marital property. If the parties have agreed on all these issues, the state will grant their divorce. If they have not agreed, the court will conduct a trial, after which the judge will decide all of these issues and dissolve the marriage.

Jurisdiction

People get divorced in the state where they reside, regardless of where they got married. In the United States, the regulation of marriage is a power of the states, and therefore each state establishes its own laws on divorce. Each state decides for itself how long one must reside before qualifying as a resident. Many years ago when divorce was hard to obtain, certain states such as Nevada made it easy to establish residence and easy to get divorced. Because one could establish residence in a few weeks, many people seeking a "quickie" divorce would fly to Reno for a month and come back divorced. The problem is that one state cannot exercise jurisdiction over property that is located in another state; so, the "quickie" divorce dissolved the marriage but often left many other issues unresolved.

Jurisdiction is generally not a problem in divorce. On occasion, it is a problem when one spouse has moved to another state, established residence, and wants to obtain the divorce in that state, believing that the laws of the new state will be more beneficial for him or her. But generally, jurisdiction is not a major issue; couples get divorced in the state in which they have been living together.

Grounds

The young couple sat in my office looking solemn. They were a Chinese couple, both in the computer programming business, who had immigrated to the United States 5 years before. When I asked how I could help them, the wife replied that she wanted a divorce from her husband. The husband quickly stated that he did not want a divorce. He said that no one in either of their families had ever divorced and that, to him, divorce was unthinkable. Looking at her, he asked, "What have I done wrong?" "You have not done anything wrong," she said. "I am just unhappy being married to you, and I want a divorce." "Happy?" he asked incredulously. "We are married. We have children. What does 'happy' have to do with it?"

Unhappiness is one of the most common reasons people state for divorce. This is a relatively new development from a historical point of view. My paternal grandparents immigrated to this country at the turn of the century and began their business with a pushcart. After some years, they were able to open a hardware store and through very hard work raise and educate three children. I try to imagine them in their store late one night and my grandmother turning to my grandfather and saying (in Yiddish), "Phillip, I'm not happy. I want a divorce!" The look she would have received would have been one of incredulity and incomprehension. "What did you say?" he would have asked. "Have you lost your mind?" And, of course, this scene would never have happened, because a marriage that was successful economically and provided for the family was more than sufficient a hundred years ago.

Although laypersons think grounds for divorce are important, in contemporary law grounds are, in fact, among the least important aspect of a divorce. Almost no divorces ever go to trial on questions of grounds. This was not always the case, however. Examining the history of divorce law—especially the issue of grounds for divorce—is illuminating, because it casts light on the institution of marriage and how it has evolved in the past century. The expectations people have about marriage have changed significantly. In particular, women's perspectives on marriage—their definition of what constitutes a "happy marriage" and what is necessary to realize this ideal–have changed and have had significant impact on the high rate of divorce.

Divorce laws have evolved and changed to keep pace with the culture. In the past, most states demanded grounds that were quasi-criminal and invariably based on fault. Only a party who had been victimized by the illicit conduct of his or her spouse could sue for divorce. The premise of a complaint for divorce was that a husband or wife had engaged in behavior that violated the covenants of marriage so egregiously that it would be unreasonable to require that person's spouse to remain in the marriage. The most common offense that could serve as grounds was infidelity. The second was desertion–that is, when a spouse left and refused to return. Depending on the state, there were other grounds as well. Extreme cruelty, addiction and alcoholism, incarceration in a jail or a mental institution, or sexual deviance have all traditionally been recognized as grounds for divorce. Divorce was serious business, because if you did establish that your spouse was guilty of some nasty behavior, the outcome of the trial could be very punitive. Alimony was tied to fault, and a woman found to be at fault received no support from her husband even if she was desperately in need. Custody of the children was usually awarded to the prevailing party, and the winning parent could literally cut the other off from the children. Perhaps because of its implicit association with deviant behavior, divorce was accompanied by social stigma, and rejection and was generally regarded as embarrassing if not humiliating.[1]

This punitive approach to divorce started to change after World War II. The modern notions of romantic love began to displace more traditional concepts of marriage, and many people–particularly women–began to demand more emotional satisfaction from their marriages. It was no longer acceptable for the spouse to be merely a good provider, monogamous, sober, and nonabusive. People expected to be happy together, and endurance was no longer the antidote for marital unhappiness. People unhappy in their marriages wanted to be able to divorce without the consent of their spouses. They wanted to be able to escape and remarry, and were increasingly unwilling to be held in the marriage against their will. Where legal statutes did not allow such divorces, people simply lied and perjured themselves to get the divorce.

By the 1970s, many state legislatures began to respond by adding new grounds to their divorce statutes. The new laws were also a reflec-

[1]See Coontz, S. (2005). *Marriage: A history*. New York: Viking Press.

tion of several other trends. One was the fact that more women were employed and not so dependent on their husbands for their livelihood. Economic independence made it easier for women to leave abusive or unsatisfying marriages. Additionally, the easy availability of reliable birth control also freed women to leave marriages and still be able to enjoy sexual relationships. Eventually, states began to pass no-fault divorce statutes that permitted people to divorce without a finding of marital wrongdoing. And by the 1980s, almost every state had adopted some form of no-fault divorce statute that permitted a divorce if the couple had lived apart for some defined period of time or if they pleaded that they were simply incompatible and could not live together.

It is important to note that the universal adoption of no-fault divorce did not *cause* people to get divorced. It simply made it easier to do. It also meant that one spouse could not hold the other in an unhappy marriage by refusing to cooperate. While there are some exceptions, today's common divorce scenario is two people who simply cannot get along–their emotional styles differ, or they cannot adapt to the practical demands and strenuous tasks of everyday family life, combined with expectations of deep emotional intimacy.

Does It Matter If the Divorce Is No-Fault or Fault-Based?

No-fault grounds usually fall into one or two categories. The majority of states provide that if spouses can prove they are incompatible or have differences that cannot be resolved, then either can obtain a divorce. The second category of no-fault grounds is some defined period of separation. If the two spouses have lived in separate homes for a period of 6 months, a year, 18 months, or 2 years (depending on the state), the court will take that fact as proof that the marriage is dead and dissolve the marriage.

In most states the consent of the other partner is not required if one partner has either fault or no-fault grounds. (One exception to this general rule is New York, in which no-fault divorce is available only when both spouses agree. But, as this is being written, the New York legislature is being pushed by the bar and judiciary of the state to modify the statute so as not to require mutual consent.) When a partner has fault grounds, the consent of the other partner is not required. There are a few states in which a finding of marital misconduct can have an impact on the outcome of a divorce. However, most states no longer take much note of allegations of marital fault. In particular, infidelity is rarely a factor when determining such matters as alimony. Even though statutes may permit the court to take such behaviors into account, few judges are willing to do so. Perhaps we have grown cynical or have simply become more sophisticated and relativistic about sexual behavior. The modern approach to divorce tends toward the view that both spouses have contributed to the demise of the marriage, even if one of the spouses has had an affair. Unfortunately, this fact has not yet fully entered the public consciousness. Many people labor under the misapprehension that they can go to court and punish their errant spouse. Most end up disillusioned when, after spending 2 years, and five figures on legal fees, they get to court and the judge is uninterested in the issue of misconduct. Grounds don't really matter. Anyone who wants a divorce can get one and can neither be stopped nor punished.

CENTRAL ISSUES IN DIVORCE

As I discussed earlier, the issues of parenting, child support, alimony, and division of marital property must be resolved in order for the husband and the wife to obtain an uncontested divorce. These are also the issues that the two must resolve in order to lead a successful life.

Why does the court want these issues to be resolved? Traditionally, marriage served as a way of organizing society. It provided for the care and supervision of children, it organized the way property was held and handed down from one generation to another, and was the basis for transmitting the values and norms of the society. Marriage established the family; a person without membership in a family was disconnected from society. Divorce was (and in some places still is) seen as a threat to this social order. If people could enter marriages and leave at will, it threatened the social fabric. So, states have always had a set of conditions to be met before a divorce is granted.

When a marriage ends, the state wants to know how the children will be cared for and supervised. The state fulfills the role of *parens patrie*, which means the parent of last resort. If a couple abandons their children, it is the state that must care for them, a task it assumes with great hesitation. Thus, the state, through its courts, wants to know who will be in charge of the children and how the divorced parents will manage the rights and duties of parental responsibility. This concern is expressed in the issues of custody, visitation, and child support.

The state has a similar concern with respect to the maintenance of the spouse. Although today, alimony can be required of wives as well as husbands, a hundred years ago alimony was strictly a matter of husbands paying ex-wives. Women generally had little independence in the economic marketplace and at the end of a marriage were not financially independent. Even when a wife was employed, her income was usually lower than her husband's and was seen as supplementary rather than primary. To some extent, this is still the case, although the gap has narrowed in recent decades. In the past, a woman's job as homemaker was always the dominant focus. So, when a marriage ended, a wife, like a child, could be left destitute and dependent on charity and the state. Alimony was a legal requirement that the court could impose to prevent the wife from becoming a ward of the state.

The third concern of the state is related to clear ownership of property. Because the family is an economic as well as a social unit, the dissolution of the family can leave questions behind about who owns what. Commerce and social order require that title to property be clear and unambiguous. You cannot buy land, businesses, or even cars if it is not clear that the person selling is the undisputed owner. So, the division of marital property is important to the state as a matter of social order, not to mention social justice. Married people have certain rights to each other's property. When you die, for example, your spouse has a right to inherit part of your estate. If you and your spouse own a house together with a right of survivorship, and then one of you dies, the other automatically receives full ownership of the house. If these rights are not terminated upon divorce, it produces confusion whenever a third party attempts to purchase the property. So, the state requires that property be divided into two bundles–his and hers–upon divorce.

Once jurisdiction, grounds, and central issues have been resolved, the court can enact the final procedural steps that lead to the formalization of divorce.

AN OVERVIEW OF THE PROCEDURE OF DIVORCE

It is 9 A.M. in the Union County Courthouse. Margie and Don Franklin wait nervously in the hall outside of Judge Green's courtroom. They are waiting for their lawyers to arrive because they are getting divorced this morning. Finally, Margie's lawyer arrives, nods hello, and goes in to let the judge's secretary know that he is there. A few minutes later, Don's lawyer arrives and also goes into the judge's chambers. Margie and Don follow the lawyers into the courtroom. A few minutes later, the lawyers emerge and announce that the judge is ready.

Although both Margie and Don feel nervous, they know that nothing surprising is about to happen. A week earlier they met with their respective lawyers to work out the final details of the settlement, which was signed 3 days ago. The settlement detailed all the necessary agreements regarding child support and alimony and division of property. Now there is nothing left to fight about. The divorce, which was filed 8 months ago, was based on the fact that they had been separated for a year. Since Margie's lawyer filed the complaint, Margie is the plaintiff and is called to the witness stand first.

After the bailiff swears her in, Margie's lawyer asks her a series of routine questions and answers, which they have rehearsed the day before.

1. Where did you live? (Margie provides the address.)
2. Did you marry Don Franklin on February 4, 1988? (Yes.)
3. Is this a copy of your marriage certificate? (Yes.)
4. Are you and your husband living together? (No.)
5. When did you separate? (A year-and-a-half ago.)
6. I show you a document titled "Separation Agreement between Don Franklin and Marjorie Franklin," dated June 4, 2003, and ask you if you recognize your signature on page 17. (Yes, that is my signature.)
7. When you signed it, did you understand it? (Yes.)
8. When you signed it, did you do so voluntarily, free of any duress? (Yes.)
9. Do you still regard it as fair, and are you requesting the court to incorporate this agreement into the judgment of divorce? (Yes.)

Following this exchange, Margie's lawyer tells the judge that he has no further questions. The judge asks Don's lawyer if she has any questions, and she says no. The judge then tells Margie to step down and orders that Don be sworn to testify.

Don takes the stand and is asked a series of questions by his lawyer almost identical to those that had been asked of Margie. He answers them accordingly and is then excused by the judge. When the parties and their lawyers are seated again, the judge speaks:

"I find that the parties were lawfully married in New Jersey on February 4, 1988, and that they separated during January 2002 and have lived apart ever since. They have established that this court has jurisdiction over the marriage and that they have satisfied the requirements of the law for a divorce by living separately and apart for more than 1 year. The parties have submitted a separation agreement, and both have testified that they signed it knowingly and voluntarily and that both regard it as fair. This court makes no independent finding with respect to the merits of that agreement and orders that it be incorporated into the judgment of divorce. Counsel will submit the appropriate judgment to me for my signature. Have a good day."

The judge signs the judgment of divorce, and the divorce is over. From start to finish, it has taken 15 minutes.

Scenes similar to this occur every business day in every county of every state in the United States. People are often surprised by the anticlimactic and perfunctory way that divorces are finalized. In some states, the procedure is done by mail, and no appearance is necessary. But the end of a divorce is bureaucratic and legal rather than emotional and dramatic. It is terse and to the point.

WHAT PRECEDES THE COURT APPEARANCE?

Margie and Don did not suddenly land in court. Before their court appearance, they went through a series of procedures, leading to a settlement.

A Negotiated Settlement

A negotiated settlement resolving issues of custody, support, and division of property usually takes place before the couple appears in court and the judge utters his declaration that the couple is divorced. Without a settlement in place, the couple is essentially asking the judge to resolve these issues by conducting a trial. Judges do not like this scenario, because their dockets are already overfilled; so, as mentioned previously, settlement is the overwhelming norm. Settlements are reached either through mediation or through negotiation between the couple's lawyers. Chapter 8 will discuss the different types of settlements and how they are negotiated.

It is possible for the couple to file for divorce prior to the signing of a settlement. Unfortunately, many if not most lawyers prefer this scenario, because they can rack up large fees preparing for a trial they know will never take place, only to reach a settlement at the courthouse door. Couples are well advised to be sure that no papers are filed with the court until a settlement has been reached.

The Pleadings

All legal proceedings of divorce–mediated or litigated, amicable or nasty–begin with the filing of a document called a *complaint for divorce.* The person who files is the plaintiff, and the other party is automatically the defendant. The complaint states the grounds on which the divorce is sought, such as separation or incompatibility. The complaint also cites the facts that the parties were married, that the marriage still exists, and that the court has jurisdiction of the divorce because the plaintiff is a bona fide resident of the state. The complaint states whether the parties have children and whether the parties have acquired assets during the marriage. The complaint ends with a "prayer for relief" in which the plaintiff tells the court what he or she wants the court to do. All complaints for divorce end with a request that the court dissolve the marriage. Any additional requests contained in the complaint depend on whether the divorce has been settled prior to the filing of the complaint. If there is a signed settlement agreement, the complaint states that fact and often requests that the court incorporate the settlement agreement into the judgment of divorce (so that it becomes part of the final court order).

It is important to note that the settlement agreement is enforceable as a contract from the day it is signed, whether the parties are divorced or not. If there is an agreement, the divorce is regarded as uncontested. The complaint for divorce will recite that there is an agreement, and the divorce moves easily through the court. The prayer for relief in a contested case is more elaborate. The plaintiff may ask the court to grant him or her custody of the children, child support, and alimony. The plaintiff also asks the court to distribute the property of the marriage between the parties.

Once the complaint has been filed with the court, a copy is

"served" on the other spouse. States differ in the manner of service. In some states the complaint can be mailed. In other states it has to be served on the defendant by the sheriff. Once the defendant has been served, he or she has a fixed amount of time, typically 30 days, to answer the complaint by filing an *answer.* In the answer, also known as a responsive pleading, the defendant admits or denies the allegations of the complaint and makes his or her own "prayers for relief" regarding custody, support, and property distribution. If the defendant fails to file an answer within the prescribed time, the plaintiff can ask the court to enter a default judgment in which the court declares the parties divorced and grants whatever relief the plaintiff has requested. In some states, if there is a signed separation agreement, the defendant frequently defaults, as there is no adverse consequence to doing so. The terms of the agreement negotiated by the parties and the court simply dissolves the marriage.

If there is an agreement, the case goes on the court's uncontested list, and the case proceeds to a final hearing. If the case is contested, it now proceeds to litigation.

Discovery

In order to either negotiate or go to trial in a divorce, each spouse needs to know the details of their own and each other's finances. In the negotiation of a typical middle-class divorce, the husband and wife simply exchange copies of their account statements and provide each other with a list of other assets. If either has questions, he or she asks the other and gets answers to those questions. If some asset, such as the house, requires an appraisal, they jointly choose an appraiser. In the sense that they are "discovering" information, we could designate this process as informal discovery.

When there is litigation, discovery is a more formal process run by the lawyers as part of preparing the case for trial. Lawyers are a suspicious lot and are loath to accept the statements of their adversaries at face value. As we will see in the next chapter, modern lawyers are also concerned about being sued for malpractice; so, many insist that full and formal discovery be conducted in every case. Even when much of that discovery turns out to be unnecessary, many lawyers argue that they cannot do their jobs responsibly without comprehensive and sometimes exhaustive investigation–which, of course, costs the couple substantial legal fees.

In a litigated divorce, every issue at dispute is subject to discovery. In order to prepare for trial, lawyers need to find out all possible details of the other party's case and to assemble the evidence they will introduce. Modern litigation, unlike what you may have seen on television, is not based on surprise. Each side is entitled to know all the details of the other's case. So, if one is going to introduce expert testimony about any issue, including custody, child support, alimony, or equitable distribution, one has to provide the other's lawyer with a copy of the expert's report. If one is going to introduce documents into evidence, one has to provide copies to the opposing counsel as well. Discovery generally takes three forms: production of documents, interrogatories, and depositions.

Production of Documents

Each side can make a demand for production of documents for any documents that can arguably be relevant to the case. Sidebar 5.1 contains a list of typical documents that the couple may be required to pro-

---

Sidebar 5.1. Documents Typically Required in Litigated Divorce

- Every bank statement for every account he or she has had in the past 5 years.
- Every check one has written and every deposit slip for 5 years.
- Every statement for every securities transaction one has made during the past 5 years.
- All tax returns for the past 5 years.
- Every statement for any debt one has incurred during the past 5 years, including copies of every loan application completed.
- All deeds one has signed or received for any real property.
- Statements for retirement and pension accounts for 5 years.
- Any appraisal of real property owned.
- A list of all assets, including household goods and jewelry.
- All employment contracts, partnership contracts, and buy–sell agreements for any business interest owned.
- The written report of any expert witness one intends to call at trial.
- Any other document that might be relevant to any fact one intends to prove at trial.

---

duce. Because even a relatively simple case can generate hundreds if not thousands of documents, document collection and review can be extremely costly.

Interrogatories

The second form of discovery involves presenting the couple with a series of written questions that must be answered in writing and sworn to as to the accuracy of the answers. Questions can include anything that might be relevant to any aspect of the case. If adultery is at issue, for example, one would be asked questions about the person with whom one is alleged to have had an affair, including when and where they met and what they did every time they met. If custody is an issue, one can be asked any question bearing on his or her role–past and present–as a parent. Each will be asked questions about one's job, career, finances, and anything else that the lawyers think relevant.

Depositions

After answers to interrogatories have been received and documents have been produced, the lawyers will then conduct depositions. A deposition is sworn testimony taken in the presence of a court reporter who prepares a transcript of the proceeding. The witness is sworn in and examined under oath. Each lawyer takes the deposition of the adversary client. At deposition, the lawyer is not limited to questions that would be admissible at trial but can ask any question–the answer to which might lead to something admissible.

The deposition of a party to divorce can easily last a day or more. Each lawyer is also entitled to take the deposition of every witness that the other will call to testify at trial. And each lawyer will take the deposition of every expert that the other will call at trial. Sidebar 5.2 contains examples of expert witnesses whose deposition might be taken in a highly contested divorce. Of course, for each expert hired by one side, an expert counterpart will be hired by the other side to contradict the testimony of the opposing expert. A complicated case can result in 30 or 40 days of depositions at a cost of $5,000 a day or more. This is where the legal bill starts to soar. All of this is in preparation for trial. But trial seldom occurs; so, the discovery becomes the background for 11th-hour settlement negotiations. And in most cases, most of the discovery was not necessary to settle the case. Although lawyers argue

Sidebar 5.2. Expert Witnesses

- Psychologists and other mental health experts testifying about the fitness of each parent.
- Forensic accountants testifying about the value of the business and the true income of a self-employed spouse.
- Economists and employment experts testifying about the employability, or lack thereof, of the spouse. (This information bears on alimony.)
- Economists testifying about the "lifestyle" and historical living standard of the spouse. (This information bears on alimony.)
- Appraisers testifying about the value of real estate, antiques, or anything else of value.
- Actuaries testifying about the value of a pension.
- Private detectives testifying about anything they were hired to investigate.

that they never know if a case will go to trial and therefore must prepare every case as if it will go to trial, much of the discovery conducted just costs a lot of money and takes a great deal of time.

In mediation only the minimum discovery that is absolutely necessary to the couple's ability to engage in informed decision making is conducted. A single neutral expert prepares expert's reports, when necessary.

Motion Practice

Depending on how crowded the local court calendar is, years can pass between the beginning and end of a contested divorce. During that time many issues can arise on which the parties do not agree. These issues have to be submitted to the court for resolution. The procedure is called a pretrial motion. Such motions can include a request that the court order temporary custody and visitation rights regarding the children, order one spouse to pay support to the other pending trial, order assets frozen, order one spouse to pay the other's legal fees, and order discovery. The court can appoint its own experts upon motion by a party and can do anything that, in the judge's broad discretion, is necessary to further the cause of justice.

Motions begin with a written application to the court made by one party that is served on the other party. The second party has a limited time to file responsive pleadings, and the court schedules a hearing. The judge can choose to hear testimony or can decide the matter based on affidavits submitted by the parties. Motions can become like minitrials and can be very expensive for the parties. In a complicated high-conflict case, a divorce can involve six or more pretrial motions. Motions can also be filed after the divorce is over. If one party believes the other is not abiding by the orders of the court, he or she will file a postjudgment motion to enforce the judgment of the court. High-conflict couples can file motions annually for years so that the litigation never ends. Motion practice is an indicator that the divorce has gone bad, and the more frequently a couple has to go to court, the more difficult their postdivorce life is likely to be.

TRIAL

Divorces that are litigated to the bitter end come to closure in a trial before the judge. The judge hears evidence and testimony and then rules on any aspect of the divorce on which the parties have not agreed. By the time a case gets to trial, most couples have agreed on custody issues and may even be in agreement on some economic issues. The judge will conduct pretrial conferences, with the lawyers attempting to settle the case without a trial. And if the judge is unable to settle all the issues, she (or he) will at least usually settle some of them and narrow the scope of trial. At the conclusion of the trial, the judge makes her findings and orders that a judgment of divorce be prepared for her signature. The parties are now divorced.

LEGAL SEPARATION

We would be remiss if we did not touch on the subject of legal separation before concluding our discussion of divorce law and procedures so as to clear up some confusion about this often misunderstood term. Legal separation can mean different things in different states. Some states, such as New York, have a formal status called "legally separated," which means that the couple has signed a separation agreement resolving all issues but is waiting for the court to dissolve the marriage. Generally these states have a prescribed time the couple must live apart before the parties can obtain the formal divorce. But legally separated means that the couple have no legal obligations to each other aside from those specified in their agreement and can act legally–sign contracts–as single people. Each is free to date others and to generally live the life of a single person. The only constraint while legally separated is that they cannot remarry until the divorce is final.

Some states such as New Jersey do not have a formal legal status called legal separation. However, a couple living separately in New Jersey and having a signed separation agreement is exactly comparable to the New York couple. The parties have the same rights and freedoms. There is just no formal designation. In some other states, "legally separated" means that the couple has agreed that their marriage is over, and each consents to the other's living apart. However, they have not yet negotiated all the terms of their final agreement. This partial separation is likely to be found in states with statutes that punish adultery. If the couple has such a partial agreement, it means that each party can date without being subject to the punitive adultery rule.

THE IMPACT OF CHANGING DIVORCE LAWS ON MARRIAGE

This chapter has laid out the basics of divorce law and how these laws evolved historically. It is clear that it's easier to obtain a divorce today than it was a century ago, and that divorce is far more common than it was then. Some social critics look at the contemporary divorce rate and worry that the institution of marriage is breaking down and disintegrating. But this is not an accurate depiction of modern marriage. Despite many changes, marriage is not going out of style. On the contrary, most people, even those who have been divorced, want to be married. Although more people are living together and more people are marrying later than they used to, about 2 million new marriages still take place every year in the United States.[2]

[2]Kreider, R. M. (2005, February). Number, timing, and duration of marriages and divorces: 2001. *Current Population Reports, P70–97*.

6 Understanding Legal Culture and the Impact of Mediation

In Chapter 5, we looked at the laws and procedures of divorce and at the historical circumstances that shaped them. Your role as a therapist goes beyond familiarity with the laws and procedures. It is equally important for you to understand the environment and culture in which these laws play out. It will be helpful to your clients if you can penetrate the mystique of the legal system, which is a subculture in itself. Not only does it have its own values and norms but also its own way of seeing the world–a perspective not shared by the rest of society. Additionally, it has its own way of socializing lawyers into its culture. Law school and subsequent employment as an "apprentice" lawyer inculcate in the new recruit the culture of the profession. If you understand this process, you will better understand the "inexplicable" behavior of your client's lawyers and will more effectively help your clients make informed decisions about the role that lawyers will play in their own divorce.

UNDERSTANDING LEGAL CULTURE AND THE ADVERSARIAL SYSTEM

Many people believe that "thinking like a lawyer" is a positive trait, in that it suggests clarity and logic. But many of the same people believe that acting like a lawyer is a negative trait, in that it suggests an amoral disregard of human welfare and what the rest of us regard as ethics. It is this contradiction that drives the public's ambivalence about lawyers.

An exploration of the problem begins with an understanding of the essential nature of the adversarial system of law and the culture it generates. Lawyers are trained to be advocates. The system operates with the assumption that when two contending adversaries rigorously present the evidence that best serves their respective clients' interests, an individual or group of individuals (judge or jury), charged with trying the facts, will be able to find the truth. Advocacy is not in itself the pursuit of truth, and therefore obtaining the truth is not the role of the advocate. Rather, that role is to persuade the truth-finder to accept a particular version of the facts that serves the advocate's client.

I recall being asked by numerous laypeople when I was in general practice how I could, in good conscience, represent a criminal defendant whom I thought or knew to be guilty. Clearly, no professional can acknowledge that he or she is in the service of evil by promoting or protecting criminal behavior. So, the answer to the question must be this: the adversarial system of justice, though flawed at times, is the best system devised for getting at the truth of an alleged wrongdoing. If I do my job and develop all the evidence that favors my client, and if my adversary similarly does his or her job and develops all the evidence that favors his or her client, we will both enable the jury to do its job—to find the truth and enact justice. My search for justice is only indirect: my participation in a broader process enables the system as a whole to do justice. Thus, justice becomes procedural rather than moral. We assume that, if we do our job and if the system works, then justice will be done. And the way to ensure that the system works is to carefully adhere to a finely drawn system of procedures that ensures fairness by denying either side an advantage in swaying the jury or the judge.

Procedural justice becomes the lawyer's substitute for the more emotionally satisfying substantive justice that occupies the layperson. So, in place of the notion that justice is about the contest for virtue, the lawyer acquires a notion that justice is about due process and an equal chance to influence the judge or jury. Lawyers become obsessed with rules—of evidence, of discovery, and of timing for bringing issues before the court. The rules include how people in the system are permitted to communicate with one another. For example, there is a carefully nurtured ritual that restricts *ex parte* communication between the judge and the attorneys and restricts communication between attorneys and the adversary client. Procedural exactitude takes the place of moral rectitude, since procedures are designed to bolster the effectiveness of the broader legal system.

But if the morality of what I do is dependent upon my participation in a larger system, it requires considerable faith in the system. If I am free to select only information that serves my client and to ignore, discredit, or even distort information that is inimical to my client's interest, then I am acting with no integrity except for the integrity of the larger system within which I participate. It is an abstract argument indeed on which to rest a moral position.

Several problems spring from this premise. The first, and perhaps most troubling, is that the practice of law and the process of litigation have changed profoundly in the past century. Remember that what saves the integrity of the system is the occurrence of a trial in which the truth is found by judge or jury. What happens to the system if we do not have the dramatic denouement of the trial? What happens if all we have is a negotiated settlement in which the two adversaries, still engaged in their sincere attempt to discredit each other's evidence, are forced to negotiate a settlement of the dispute? Is justice still done? Is the truth still found? Or, does the stronger party simply wear down the weaker party until resistance is impractical?

These questions are rooted in social and historical reality. In the past hundred years, the incidence of trials has decreased so much that trials are now the exception rather than the rule. About 85–90% of criminal matters are resolved by plea bargains. About 95–97% of all civil suits are resolved by negotiated settlement. And in some areas of the law, such as divorce, the negotiated settlement rate can approach 99%, with less than 1% of cases going to trial. It is common wisdom that it is better to negotiate a settlement than to risk the uncertainties associated with going to trial. I could even argue that, given the overwhelming norm of settlement, trials have become the pathological exception rather than the rule. This is especially the case with divorce. In my experience, divorces do not go to trial unless at least one or more clients or lawyers is just plain crazy.

However, the myth that legal cases end in a trial is constantly reinforced by popular culture. The proliferation of books, movies, television programs, and media coverage of celebrity trials suggests that in American culture the trial has displaced the movie western as the ultimate soap opera. That few lawsuits actually work this way has not yet tarnished the public's fantasy version of the legal system. Even more disturbingly, the norm of negotiated settlement has not yet penetrated legal education in significant ways. Almost all legal education continues to be devoted to reviewing, learning, and discussing appellate cases. But what are law students really studying? To get into the casebooks, a suit must first go to trial. Today, that limits us to less than 5%

of the litigated universe. Then the case has to be appealed, and this further reduces the sample to a tiny percentage of all litigation. The actual number of cases that make their way into the legal textbooks is even smaller, because many cases do not get published unless their appeal goes to the highest court. So, the result is legal textbooks that reflect perhaps 1 case in 2,000. These published cases are representative only of the most aberrant and highly conflicted sample of the legal universe. And it is this skewed, unrepresentative sample that constitutes most of the legal education. Legal educators defend the system by telling us that this is the only way to train the student to think like a lawyer. Perhaps it is. But therein may lie the problem.

Legal Education as Acquired Disability

Law school relies on mystique to win the allegiance of its new recruits. The holy grail of law school is to "think like a lawyer." To that end, law school classes follow a time-honored tradition of public recitation by students while being grilled by the professor. The student is expected to identify all the legal issues raised by the case and to be able to argue for and against each side by mustering those facts and legal principles that would support one side or the other. The game is played by having the student answer one question and then having the professor ask a question that confounds the answer given, while raising another contradictory possibility. Correctly executed, this method continually demonstrates any given problem has no single answer but rather a multitude of possible answers.

The skill of thinking like a lawyer raises two concerns. First is the sharp analytic skill that enables the lawyer to compare one situation to another and dissect out the tiniest distinguishing characteristic. The distinction is used to argue that this case is really different from another virtually identical case in which the ruling was adverse to the client represented. But this is not just a matter of sharp thinking. It also promotes the proposition that advocacy is the ultimate value-free profession. By learning the value of arguing each side with equal fervor, the student is gradually weaned from the naive notions about truth that he or she came in with. This weaning process is reinforced by public embarrassment of students who fail to meet the professor's expectations. The heroes of the class are those students who are meticulously prepared and verbally equipped to argue forcefully, but who can turn on a dime to argue the other way when asked. Hard work and a facile tongue are the necessary equipment for the lawyer-hero. By contrast, the student who continues to cling to the notion that there really is truth and that justice requires its explication becomes the class goat who is counseled that maybe he or she would find a more congenial surrounding in social work school.

The second concern is that legal thinking is the antithesis of scientific thinking and inquiry. The scientific method demands evidence-based conclusions, where data are gathered and analyzed rigorously and serve the ultimate goal of truth. The conclusion emerges from the data and may actually disprove the original hypothesis. By contrast, a lawyer starts with a commitment to persuasion that overrides the commitment to truth. Facts are cited to support a preexisting conclusion—the position of the client. The result is indifference to data and to statistics as a way of understanding things. This is reflected in the fact that there are practically no statistical data about the outcomes of legal representation. In fact, few lawyers have ever studied statistics or acquired the insight that an understanding of sampling theory can impart in thinking about policy or other phenomena. So, even though almost all lawsuits are settled, there is little or no research about the settlement norms that influence the settlement negotiations. This means that each lawyer relies on his own experience, plus whatever anecdotal information is acquired from other lawyers. A research tradition in which information is systematically gathered for dispassionate analysis is lacking in the legal intellectual tradition.

Law and Divorce

It is in the field of divorce that the image of lawyers finds its most odious expression and where legal training is most disabling and counterproductive. Divorce lawyers have a terrible reputation among the lay public for being cynical, indifferent to suffering, and greedy for ever larger legal fees. There are, of course, divorce lawyers who do not fit this stereotype. But in over 20 years in the field, I have met more who do conform to this image than those who defy it.

It is not that divorce law attracts amoral people. In fact, some of the most sensitive of students I met in law school were attracted to "family law," where they thought they could help families. The problem lies in the juxtaposition of the adversarial culture onto the changing needs of families. During the past 50 years, divorce law has evolved to reflect the changing perceptions of marriage. When divorce was still a quasi-criminal proceeding and was based exclusively on the wrongdoing of one spouse, there was a good fit with the adversarial system, which is organized around the finding of wrongdoing.

But the fit began to fail as the concepts of marriage and divorce evolved in the 20th century to reflect yearnings for intimacy and happiness rather than retribution for wrongful behavior. Today, roughly 50% of marriages end in divorce.[1] Thus, divorce can no longer be regarded as socially deviant behavior based on the wrongdoing of one or the other spouse.

One would think that no-fault divorce law would make divorce easier to obtain; but getting a divorce has become more difficult and complicated. Legislatures have tinkered with more complicated schemes for dividing property, it has become common for a divorce to take 3 or more years and to generate legal fees well into six figures. When it gets out of hand, divorce supports legions of accountants, appraisers, actuaries, psychotherapists, and social workers of all descriptions. Divorce has become a multibillion-dollar business.

A second important change is that most divorces are resolved by negotiation rather than trial. The judge is seldom the decision maker. Instead, the lawyer, as negotiator, has become more central and more intrusive. And there is little in the training of lawyers that prepares them for this role. As the lawyer becomes the surrogate for the client, he or she assumes responsibility for negotiating a settlement that shapes the lives of an entire family. Yet, few lawyers know much about family dynamics or emotional processes. And few lawyers understand how the negotiating positions they take affect the way the clients feel about each other. So, by the time the lawyers finish with their posturing and threats, there is a negotiated agreement in place, but the relationship between the spouses is so poisonous that it negates cooperation in the future. Consequently, the process of getting divorced has as much adverse impact on divorcing families as the fact of the divorce itself. And when confronted by the emotional carnage they produce, divorce lawyers deny that their actions have anything to do with it. Rather, they insist, it is the inherent irrationality of divorcing people that accounts for all the bitterness of divorce.

[1]Norton, A., & Miller, L. (1992, October). Marriage, divorce, and remarriage in the 1990's. *Current Population Reports, P23–180.*

CASE STUDY: JULIE AND STAN

After a 20-year marriage, Julie and Stan were divorcing. Things had been getting worse for years, with a gradual coldness setting in between the two. The couple's son Michael, age 15, had noticed that his parents rarely talked at dinner, and he often found excuses to be elsewhere at suppertime. As Julie and Stan became more distant from each other, each coped in his or her own way with the growing sense of loneliness. Stan threw himself into his work. He was a manager for a software company that was launching several new products. He made his job his top priority and no longer resisted the temptation to schedule evening meetings and projects. He found companionship and purpose at work that distracted him from the distress he felt when he went home. He still hoped that Julie would come around and realize that she really had a good husband. He loved Julie but felt he could never make her happy. The last sexual encounter between the couple had taken place 9 months ago, and he missed Julie's sexual companionship. Now, Julie usually went to sleep in the guest room.

Julie was also very lonely. She was a teacher but did not find much companionship at school. Until the past few years, she had devoted herself to the family, ferrying Michael around after school and maintaining a warm and inviting home. But recently Michael had morphed into a typical adolescent who wanted little contact with his parents. Michael spent most of his time on school, sports, and with his friends. For the first time in many years, Julie found life unsatisfying and boring. She had pretty much given up on her relationship with Stan. He had refused her many requests that they go into couple therapy, telling her that he didn't believe that some shrink could do what they could not. He told her that if she stopped moping around, regained her sense of fun, and took some interest in sex, they would be fine. She despaired of ever understanding what she needed and had no interest in trying to find out. Recently she had begun to flirt with a long-held taboo–that maybe she and Stan needed to divorce.

One week when she was feeling particularly down, a friend of hers suggested that the two of them go away for a weekend of square dancing, which was her friend's passion. Julie agreed and told Michael and Stan to fend for themselves for the weekend, because she was going off with her friend Erica. From the time the two arrived at the resort where the meeting was being held, Julie had a great time. People were friendly and cheerful, and before long she was enjoying herself. Toward the middle of the first evening, she realized that she knew one of the men who was there, Larry, who was in fact the first boy she had ever dated many years before. The two of them reminisced for hours and quickly rekindled the spark they had shared 30 years earlier. He was divorced and living in a city about an hour away. He was still handsome and was gentle and attentive to her. By the end of the weekend she was smitten, and the two exchanged phone numbers. She had told him that she was married but feared that her marriage was not going to survive for long. There was to be another square dance gathering in a month, and the two agreed to meet there again.

During the month the two emailed back and forth frequently. Julie was delighted to have someone who was really interested in communicating with her and who was open with his feelings. It made her feel a little guilty though, and she didn't mention it to Stan. When she and Larry met again a month later the relationship bloomed quickly, and by the end of the first day the two were in bed together. Although she continued to feel guilty, Julie was ecstatic. She decided that it wasn't fair to have missed affection and passion for so long and that it was time to get a divorce. That Sunday night when she got home, she told Stan that the two of them needed to talk. She said that things had been bad for too long between them and that his refusal to go into therapy over the past year had convinced her that it was hopeless. She was unhappy, he was unhappy, and it clearly was doing no good for Michael. So, she had decided that the two of them should consider divorce.

Stan was stunned. Although he acknowledged that things had been bad for a long time, he had resigned himself to the status quo and had not even considered divorce. Why not wait a while until at least Michael had graduated from high school? In the meantime they would see how things went, and maybe he would reconsider his objection to therapy. But Julie was no longer interested. "There's nothing left, Stan. There's nothing to work with. I don't love you anymore, and we just don't have a marriage to work on. It has eroded and dribbled away. It's too late, and I don't want to spend any more time on it. Let's do it decently, but let's do it."

Stan was so blindsided by Julie's clarity that he didn't say much. He said that he would think about it and went to watch television. After thinking about things the next day, Stan told her that he thought it was a mistake but recognized that if she was insistent he couldn't stop her. Stan then retreated into moody silence. "Why now?" he thought, "Why so suddenly?" He wondered if Julie was having an affair. Stan was an accomplished computer expert and had little trouble hacking into Julie's email. There, plain as could be, was the confirmation of his suspicion. He read all the exchanges between Julie and Larry and concluded that she simply used their marital unhappiness as an excuse but was really leaving him for another man. That evening he confronted Julie with his evidence. Julie was incensed that he had violated her privacy and was equally angry that he was blaming everything on her affair with Larry. "I have lived through your withdrawal for years. I have suffered your insensitivity and your stupid refusal to do anything to help the marriage. By the time I even met Larry, our marriage was totally dead. How can you be so blind? You just won't take responsibility!"

The next day, Stan consulted a lawyer who had represented a friend of his. "What are my rights?" he demanded after recounting his story. The lawyer, Marian Boone, replied that according to the law of New Jersey a judge might consider the adultery as a factor mitigating against alimony but that it was discretionary and some judges would not consider it important. She advised Stan that if the judge was unimpressed by the fact of adultery, Stan would probably be ordered to pay Julie alimony for at least 7–10 years. However, she implied, it was worth attempting to introduce the adultery, since there was a good chance that Judge Gibbs—known to be an ultraconservative "family values" man—would probably take Julie's affair into account. "Either way, it won't hurt your case and might even help," Marian said. She also suggested that Stan would win a custody fight if his son told the judge that he wanted to stay with his father. If that happened, Stan might be able to stay in the house until the son graduated from high school, avoid selling the house, and split the equity with Julie once that happened.

THE COMPONENTS OF THE LAWYER'S ADVICE

Before clients hire lawyers, they need to think about how they want to use the lawyers. Lawyers offer to provide a number of services, but clients may not be well served by all such services. Let us deconstruct the advice that Stan's lawyer gave him.

Advice about the Law

The first role of the lawyer in divorce is to educate clients about the law of divorce and suggest how it will apply to them. For example, Stan's lawyer advised him that in New Jersey adultery can be a factor but not necessarily a bar to a woman's right to receive alimony. The lawyer also explained how state law applies to other issues that will have to be resolved, such as child custody, child support, and distribution of property. Clients usually ask their lawyers to tell them about their "legal rights." But lawyers can answer questions about legal rights only to a degree. That is, a lawyer can state his or her opinion about how a particular client's legal rights might be interpreted by a judge. But because of the nature of divorce law, the lawyer usually cannot prognosticate with precision or certainty. With the exception of child support, which is subject to federally mandated guidelines, divorce statutes generally establish broad parameters within which judges are supposed to decide cases. For example, when parents cannot agree on custody, the judge is directed to decide in the "best interests of the child." But how a given judge will decide in a particular case is subject to considerable speculation. Your client's lawyer may be able to tell if your client has a strong or a weak case but can seldom tell with any certainty whether he or she will prevail.

This adds a complication to what we call legal advice, because it has the lawyer speculating not about the law itself but about how the law may be applied by a particular judge. It is in this area that the client must be very careful, because lawyers frequently are wrong in their predictions. Thus, Stan's lawyer may be of the opinion that a judge would find Julie guilty of moral turpitude, conclude that she is morally unfit to be the primary parent of the child, and award custody of the child to Stan. And Judge Gibbs, who is socially conservative, might do just that. But on the other hand, Judge Smith, who is not so conservative, might decide that Julie's affair–although technically adultery–really has nothing to do with her moral fitness and may refuse to even consider it when making a decision. And even Judge Gibbs might overcome his social disapproval of Julie and award her custody if Stan is particularly unappealing or Julie is particularly attractive. All of these "nonrational" factors play a role and detract from a lawyer's ability to prognosticate accurately. On innumerable occasions I have seen two experienced divorce lawyers look at the same case and predict with certainty totally opposite results if the case goes to trial. So, your client's lawyer can tell her what the law is and predict how it *might* be applied. But one needs to retain some degree of skepticism.

Advice about Negotiation Strategy

The analysis becomes even murkier when we consider that there is a very low probability that any case will ever go before a judge for resolution and instead will be settled by negotiation. So, in most cases, the lawyer's prediction of what a judge might or might not do is irrelevant on a practical level. Rather, it is intended as a backdrop for negotiations. Most lawyers will argue in settlement negotiations that the settlement should reflect what a judge would do if the case went to trial. In fact, this becomes the primary subject lawyers argue about in negotiations. So, Stan's lawyer would try to convince Julie's lawyer that because Julie had engaged in adultery she should not get alimony. In fact, she should settle for little or no alimony because Judge Gibbs, who would probably hear the case, would rule that way. And then Julie's lawyer would argue that the marriage was already dead when Julie had her one-night affair and that she was desperately lonely after living for 20 years with a cold fish like Stan. No judge—even the conservative Judge Gibbs—would hold it against her. Therefore, the lawyer would argue, Julie's alimony should not be affected by her affair.

The actual impact of these arguments on the settlement negotiations might be affected by several other unpredictable factors, such as how effective each lawyer is as a negotiator. Although almost all lawyers regard themselves as good negotiators, many are only mediocre, and more than a few are poor negotiators. Unfortunately, one has no way of knowing in advance whether a given lawyer is also a skilled negotiator. A second factor is the degree to which either spouse wants to settle the matter and be done with it. The spouse who is more eager for closure may make concessions that he or she would not otherwise make. On the other hand, if one lawyer has stoked his or her client's anger and that spouse craves the drama of a courtroom trial, he or she may be less willing to concede anything in negotiation. A lawyer's willingness to go to trial may also be a factor in the way he or she encourages the client to agree or not to agree to negotiations. Some lawyers are more belligerent than others. Some value amicable settlements and prefer to settle rather than go to trial. Some lawyers always practice brinkmanship and never settle until the last minute. Finally, sad to say, some lawyers are hungrier or greedier than others and won't let a case settle until they have milked the maximum fee. In every town and city there are at least a few members of the divorce bar who are well known to their colleagues for this unfortunate proclivity. Of course, these lawyers pride themselves on their fierce advocacy style and believe that they are actually serving the interests of their clients by waging a war of attrition even though doing so results in large fees to the client. And again, regrettably, laypeople often succumb to the myth that by getting the meanest, baddest lawyer in town they will acquire an advantage, when in reality doing so usually leads them to the predator types. The predator lawyer's first meal is usually his or her own client.

Much of what passes for legal advice is not information about the law but advice from the lawyer about how to pursue a competitive advantage over the spouse. In the case of Stan, the lawyer advised him that his son would likely want to live with him and that he would probably be able to remain in the house. To Stan, eager for any advantage over Julie, this "advice" was welcome and shaped his perspectives of what his "rights" were. What you need to remember is that these predictions of outcomes by your client's lawyer may not be accurate and may be influenced by many philosophical, stylistic, and economic characteristics of the lawyer, few of which will be known to the client.

Philosophical Advice

When Stan's lawyer counseled him to file suit and attempt to deny alimony to Julie, she was not only giving legal advice but also giving philosophical advice. That is, she made a value judgment that the legal maneuver to deprive Julie of support was *worth* doing. Let's assume that the lawyer was correct in her prediction that Judge Gibbs will deprive Julie of alimony. What will happen then? We can predict that Julie will be bitter. We can also predict that the couple's son will be affected by that bitterness and that the legacy of anger generated will last for a long time. When Michael graduates from high school or college, when he gets married or has children, Stan and Julie will be unable to come together with any sense of goodwill toward each other. Julie's anger at what she regards as unjust treatment by Stan will be communicated to Michael, who will feel torn between his parents. He will be confused and upset by his father's depiction of his mother as immoral and will realize that his parents can no longer have civil or cooperative communication even when his needs are at stake. These are the completely predictable outcomes if Stan follows his lawyer's advice. I have never been impressed by the collective wisdom of lawyers. Clients should be wary when lawyers, in the guise of legal advice, try to steer them unduly in regard to philosophical decisions. By "philosophical" I mean those decisions that are guided by the value preferences of the lawyer rather than a clear understanding of the consequences. In assuming a philosophical perspective, some lawyers are particularly handicapped by their own culture. Martin Seligman, a noted researcher on cognition and depression, reports that lawyers are the only professional group in which pessimism as a personal style is correlated with professional success.[2] Lawyers also have the highest divorce rate, suicide rate, and incidence of depression and professional dissatisfaction rate of any of the professions.[3] This is hardly an endorsement of the typical practitioner's mastery of life's mysteries and the intricacies of human relationships. Moreover, the training of lawyers teaches them a concept of client representation in which the object is to shift as much of the cost and as much of the risk to the other guy's client as possible. But it is a philosophy that disables them from assessing the needs of their client's family as it adjusts to the changes required by divorce. So, the win-at-any-cost viewpoint, though appealing from a legal perspective, can be devastating to their client's long-term interests.

Advice on Family Dynamics

Because the legal strategies adopted by lawyers have such an impact on the ability of the family to adapt to divorce, one would think that divorce lawyers are knowledgeable about family dynamics, child development, and the psychology of conflict. In my 25 years of experience with thousands of lawyers, I have not found this to be true. The greatest obstacle to such understanding is the legal culture's discomfort with the nonrational parts of life. Rational behavior refers to those of our actions driven by an understanding of our interests. Irrational behavior is that which is driven by self-destructive impulses. In my opinion, most human behavior is nonrational–that is, behavior driven by feelings. Nonrational behavior may have either destructive or constructive consequences, but the important fact is that most behavior is driven by feelings and emotions. What this means is that a fully developed understanding of emotional life is absolutely critical to understanding complex human behavior and to intervening in an intelligent manner. And it is the recognition of the emotional side of life that legal education deliberately screens out.

[2]Seligman, M. (2002). *Authentic happiness*. New York: Free Press.

[3]Ibid.

So, when it comes to giving advice on how to achieve sound *family* objectives, lawyers have little professional training that is helpful. Most lawyers do not give good advice about child custody issues and tend to exacerbate rather than calm their clients' fears. Stan's lawyer, for example, rushed in to suggest that Michael would want to live with Stan and that it would be advantageous for the two of them to remain in the house—all without delving into the actual nature of the relationship between Michael and his parents.

And few lawyers define their objectives in terms of what helps a family to thrive over time. Your client's lawyer is concerned with how to get him or her the most of what he or she thinks the client wants. Stan's lawyer wants to help him pay the least support even if that has an adverse effect on his son and wife. The lawyer wants to get him the best deal on property distribution even if that has an adverse effect as well. That lawyer's job is to shift as much of the risk, cost, and dislocation as possible to the client's spouse. That is the legal advocate's job by definition, but that job description is notoriously shortsighted and unable to anticipate the long-term effects on your client's emotional welfare or that of his or her family.

Stan was impressed with the advice given him by his lawyer. He didn't want the divorce, but he concluded that since it was being forced on him, he ought to strike first and get the best deal he could. By showing Julie how tough he could be, he would certainly improve his bargaining position, and if they couldn't reach a settlement, at least he would have an advantage in court. So, he told the lawyer to go ahead and file for the divorce, alleging that Julie had committed adultery and asking the court for custody of Michael and the award of child support from Julie. His lawyer asked for a $5,000 retainer and directed Stan to empty the joint bank accounts and to move the investment account into accounts in his name alone. The lawyer told him that, in her experience, if Stan didn't get there first, Julie would, and then Stan would be at her mercy. So, Stan followed his lawyer's advice, paid the retainer, and moved the money. The lawyer filed a complaint for divorce and directed the sheriff to serve a copy of the complaint upon Julie.

Stan said nothing to Julie about the complaint's being filed. He figured that the shock value would help bring Julie to her senses and plead for peace. Julie was indeed shocked when the sheriff came to the school where she was teaching to serve the complaint. She was absolutely stunned by the allegations of the complaint and couldn't believe that Stan had done this to her. But the shock did not have the effect Stan had hoped for. Instead, it backfired against him. Within a short time her surprise turned to rage. She called her friend Beverly and told her what had happened, and Beverly gave her the name of her brother's divorce lawyer who was reputed to be one of the toughest lawyers in town. The same afternoon, Julie discovered that the money had been moved and that she had no access to the family's savings. This frightened her even more. So, she called the lawyer and pleaded with his secretary to fit her in for an emergency appointment. The following morning, she took the complaint she had received to the lawyer Marvin Mason. Mason advised her that she would have to file an answer to Stan's complaint. He also advised her to file a counterclaim that alleged that Stan was guilty of extreme cruelty toward her and citing at length all the details of Stan's cruel behavior. In her counterclaim she would ask for custody of Michael, child support, alimony, and distribution of the marital assets. She would also ask the court to order Stan to put the family savings back in the joint accounts, for an order forbidding Stan from making any unilateral disposition of assets, and an order of temporary support for her and Michael. Mason asked for a $7,500 retainer and said he could not start the case without it. But because the savings were all in Stan's control, she would have to go to friends or family to borrow the money until the court ordered Stan to put back the money he had taken.

Julie went home and called several friends, her brother, and her sister. They were infuriated by Stan's outrageous actions, but none of them had ready cash. In desperation, Julie called her parents, who agreed to lend her the money. She got a check from her father and paid Mason. He filed the answer and counterclaim and asked the court for an emergency hearing. The war had begun.

LEGAL ADVICE REVISITED

We have described four components of legal advice. The formal training of lawyers incorporates only the first, an understanding of the law. Some lawyers acquire good negotiation skills through experience, and a few even take courses to develop negotiation skills and techniques. As to philosophical expertise, some lawyers acquire some wisdom as they mature, but many clearly do not. The same applies to psychological advice. Here I regard most lawyers as seriously handicapped by their training, and I have met very few who have anything approaching an adequate appreciation of what promotes families' emotional health.

It is important that clients consult with lawyers. It is equally important that they not grant a lawyer greater authority than is actually warranted by the skills and wisdom of that particular lawyer. As soon as one gets beyond advice on the law, skepticism should grow as the lawyer proposes to make strategic philosophical, psychological, and negotiation judgments about how one proceeds. The lawyer's advice in these areas is shaped more by his personality and culture than by his expertise.

LIMITING THE ROLE OF THE LAWYER

By now you are aware that the less contact had by the client with the judicial system, the better off he or she will be. Similarly, the less contact they have with their lawyers, within certain parameters, the better off they are as well. Clients should use their lawyers to learn as much as possible about the legal rules that apply to their divorce. They should have their lawyers teach them about the law as it applies to parenting, support issues, and property issues. If there are technical issues, the lawyer may advise about tax implications or what valuation methods should be applied to the assets. They should have the lawyer advise them, as background information only, what norms might be applied if negotiations were to fail and the matter went to court. But they should use their lawyers primarily as teachers about the law so that they can stay in charge of the negotiations with each other. That is the chief objective. Moreover, they should hear their lawyers' opinions about matters that are essentially strategic, philosophical, or psychological–so long as they retain their skepticism about the validity of that lawyer's opinions. But on the psychological matters, they should also consult a good therapist; and on philosophical matters, they should find someone they regard as wise and listen.

MEDIATION

Since lawyers play an important role in the divorce process and this process is transacted in the legal arena, pessimism can arise on the part of both therapists and clients regarding the prospect of reaching the desired goal–a good divorce. It is reassuring to know that there is an alternative approach to divorce: mediation. Mediation provides the couple with the tools and skills necessary to craft the building blocks of a good divorce. Therapists can play a crucial role in encouraging clients who are contemplating divorce to seek mediation rather than litigation.

What Is Mediation?

Mediation had been around for thousands of years. In traditional societies, mediation was the common and expected way to resolve disputes. The village elder or wise man would help disputants negotiate an amicable resolution. Religious and community leaders have long been relied on to mediate in communities. A mediator does not make decisions for people in disputes, but rather facilitates the communication of the disputants. When people disagree, it is easy for their emotions to interfere with their ability to engage in constructive discussion and negotiation. The anger that arises when one person feels wronged, falsely accused, or criticized results in indignation and an impulse to retaliate and punish. Unless people find a way to manage their feelings, discussion deteriorates into an exchange that is unpleasant and unproductive. But when the discussion is guided and contained, most people can talk out the disagreement and find mutually acceptable resolution. That is traditionally the role of the mediator.

The mediator uses the mutual needs of the parties to establish his or her authority. The mediator provides a safe environment for discussion and imposes rules of conduct that ensure that the discussion stays on track and does not deteriorate into personal attacks. When necessary, the mediator establishes the agenda for the meeting and helps harness the creativity and knowledge of the parties in a search for amicable resolution. Mediation is a craft–part learned technique and part art. Like a good therapist, a good mediator has personal characteristics that command respect, establish rapport, and provide a calming influence. And, like therapy, mediation is usually a voluntary process (unlike binding arbitration). Mediators have no power other than the power to withdraw when a party to the dispute refuses to cooperate.

The History of Divorce Mediation

The divorce mediation movement is about 25 years old, but it has acquired additional momentum during the past 10 years. It began during the late 1970s with a group of reform-minded lawyers who were appalled by the carnage they were witnessing in the divorce courts. They began to collaborate with psychologists and family therapists to find a more decent and humane way to facilitate divorce. The mediation movement began in a few states, most notably New Jersey and Minnesota, and by the early 1980s had become a national movement. The premises were simple. These pioneers recognized that, although almost all divorces were resolved with a negotiated settlement, that settlement came only after years of litigation in which both sides prepared for a trial that only rarely occurred. With the settlement as the incidental but inevitable by-product of preparing for trial, couples were put through a process that served as a meat grinder for whatever was left of family cooperation. They reasoned that, if the case were going to settle eventually anyway, why not redesign the system to pursue settlement at the *beginning* of the divorce rather than at the end? Instead of having the couple surrender all power to an adversarial process, why not keep the husband and wife in control and facilitate their ability to negotiate and reach a settlement that they would themselves craft? That was the beginning of divorce mediation.

What came out of these discussions 25 years ago was a movement that at present includes thousands of practitioners and would-be practitioners around the country. At present, the Association for Conflict Resolution, the largest national organization, has thousands of members. However, the development of the divorce mediation movement, from its inception and early roots to the established entity it is today, was not a smooth or easy process. Mediation was initially received with great hostility by the organized bar associations. The notion that one professional could help two parties negotiate their own settlement of a conflict violated many tenets of the legal culture. Many lawyers painted vivid pictures in their minds of a horde of unqualified mediators promoting unfair settlements that robbed innocent people of their rights and produced unfair results. When I started offering divorce mediation in New Jersey in 1979, the bar association grumbled that I ought to be disbarred, because mediation, in their opinion, constituted a violation of the ethics rules of legal practice. It took a long time and great controversy within the profession to win a grudging acceptance for divorce mediation.

Mediation not only violated the cultural norms of the legal profession but also represented a serious economic threat. Divorce was the bread-and-butter income producer for most small law firms, and a process that could reduce legal fees by as much as 90% was clearly unwelcome.

But, over 25 years later, mediation has become a permanent part of the divorce landscape. Lawyers as a group have not endorsed it, but the mental health professions have generally been enthusiastic. Most of the referrals to divorce mediators still come from therapists, although an increasing number of referrals come from satisfied clients. Therapists like it because it reduces the negative consequences of divorce. It enables families to reorganize at less emotional and financial cost; so, it minimizes the impact of the divorce on couples and their children. Successfully done, mediation allows people to move on with their lives and curbs the type of chronic conflict that haunts many families who have endured conventional divorce.

Mediation and Risk

Divorce mediation is essentially a no-risk proposition. Nothing is binding until the agreement reached by the parties has been set forth in a contract prepared or reviewed by the parties' attorneys. People commit to mediation one hour at time and can withdraw if they believe it is not working. Most mediators charge per session and do not collect retainers. So, if the clients do not want to continue with mediation after three or four sessions, they have lost very little time or money. They can always revert to a conventionally negotiated or litigated divorce. But if mediation does work, it usually spells the difference between a bad divorce and a good divorce. I regard it as the first choice for almost all couples. If one of the spouses is violent, crazy, addicted, or so oppositional that cooperative discussion is impossible, then mediation is not the answer. But, for more than 90% of all couples, mediation is an appropriate choice.

With Lawyers or Without?

Divorce mediation originally developed as a process that was done without the parties' lawyers in the room. The model of mediation that has generally been practiced is one in which the couple have advisory or consulting lawyers with whom they talk whenever they, or the mediator, feel that they need a consultation. Lawyers are used as advisors and counselors rather than surrogates and do not attend the sessions because that would defeat the purpose of keeping the couple in charge. Additionally, on a practical level, it is too difficult to schedule meetings with two divorcing individuals and three busy professionals. It is also too expensive because three professionals are being paid instead of one. An important goal of mediation is for the couple to learn a new way of talking to each other so they can continue to communicate and cooperate around the children well after the divorce is over. When lawyers dominate the discussion, it defeats the integrity of that process.

The only circumstances in which lawyers should be present in a mediation session are when one or both of the parties is so impaired that he or she cannot carry on a fruitful discussion. I have invited lawyers to participate in mediation sessions when there have been allegations of domestic violence or addiction or when one of the parties is so timid that he or she is unable to participate fully. Lawyer-dominated mediation is preferable to litigation but is much less productive than mediation in which the clients do the talking.

Court-Mandated Mediation

As mediation became more accepted, two developments occurred. Courts came under pressure to make the advantages of mediation available to litigants; and many lawyers sought a way to reinvolve themselves in divorces by co-opting a process that had reduced their centrality. The result is court-annexed mediation, which barely resembles the real thing. Many courts have set up programs that are called "divorce mediation" but lack any of the advantages of real mediation. First, lawyers are usually present and do most of the talking. Second, the mediation is ordered late in the case after the damage has already been done by the adversarial process—typically, when litigation is well under way and the parties have already been polarized. Third, it is usually a one-time event that does not afford the mediator time to establish trust and rapport with the clients, which he or she could not do in any event because the lawyers are doing the talking. Finally, the quality of the mediators is generally poor, because they are either unpaid volunteers or poorly trained and poorly qualified court personnel. Because most cases settle anyhow as the trial draws near, court-annexed mediation has often become a waste of time and money for the clients. It just creates another billing event for the lawyers and accomplishes little else.

COLLABORATIVE LAW

Before we leave the subject of legal culture and its impact on the divorce process, we should touch briefly upon another alternative to destructive litigation–collaborative law. A few years ago some lawyers began to advertise a novel approach to negotiating agreements. Each client would be represented by a lawyer, as in conventional divorce. The difference was that each lawyer would promise not to begin any action in the court until settlement was reached. Moreover, each lawyer agreed that, if at any point the parties were deadlocked and wanted to go to court, the lawyers would resign, requiring the clients to hire new lawyers. The premise was that the refusal to go to court would remove a threatening tone that often accompanies lawyer-driven negotiation. This would promote more of a problem-solving approach and an amicable atmosphere. Additionally, the cooperative posture would make it possible to choose neutral appraisers, accountants, and actuaries to value assets such as businesses and pensions.

Although collaborative law garnered some media attention, I am not aware that many people use it. The chance of having to start all over with another lawyer if things don't work out dissuades some prospective clients. The biggest disadvantage from my perspective is that it maintains the lawyer as the central figure in the process. When lawyers negotiate on behalf of clients, clients tend to be passive and don't learn to communicate directly. It lacks the advantages of mediation and retains the clunky necessity of scheduling around two lawyers' busy schedules. If your clients want to have a cooperative divorce, I recommend mediation. Perhaps for the few clients who cannot mediate but want something more cooperative, collaborative lawyers might be worth a try.

THE ROLE OF SKILLED PROFESSIONALS

The success of any process depends on the skills of its practitioners. An inept mediator can inadvertently sabotage a couple's chances of using mediation effectively to facilitate communication and reach a settlement with which they are comfortable, and can unwittingly drive the couple into the waiting arms of lawyers. The next chapter looks at several different types of settlements–both mediated and litigated–and how to help your clients choose the lawyers and mediators that most effectively serve their needs.

7 Helping Your Clients Use Lawyers and Mediators Effectively

Now that you understand the laws and procedures surrounding divorce, the pitfalls of the legal system, and the process of mediation, you are in a better position to advise your clients about negotiating a settlement, choosing lawyers and mediators, and using these professionals to maximum advantage. This chapter will expand your understanding of the role that mediators and lawyers play in the divorce process and will provide the tools to help your clients make informed choices.

TYPES OF SETTLEMENTS

To help you get oriented, I would like to review the different routes to settlement possible between divorcing couples and to look at which particular route seems most appropriate for your clients. This will inform their decision of whether mediated or lawyer-negotiated settlement is the best fit and, if so, what type of professional to select.

Lawyer-Negotiated Litigated Settlement

This is the most conventional scenario. Each party hires a lawyer, and the lawyers talk to each other, with clients communicating only to their respective lawyers. In most cases the lawyers disagree with each other and resort to filing pleadings in the court so that they can litigate the matter under the supervision of the court. Typically, they file a complaint immediately, prior to negotiating an agreement. They conduct discovery, engage in pretrial motions, and generally prepare for trial. Then, on the eve of trial, they negotiate the settlement.

Collaborative Law Nonlitigated Settlement

This scenario also relies on lawyers as central but makes the negotiation of the agreement the primary goal, with litigation reserved only as an act of desperation. There is an implicit agreement among the lawyers and the clients that they will not go to court and will do whatever is necessary to negotiate successfully. And if during the negotiations the client decides to file in court, the lawyer is committed to resigning. Obviously, this collaborative law scheme works only when both clients retain lawyers with the same commitment.

Mediated Settlement

The third alternative is a mediated divorce in which the clients retain control, are central to the negotiation process, and use lawyers only as advisors when they need legal advice. In mediation, a trained mediator facilitates the negotiation between the two spouses and provides the leadership necessary for productive discussions and reaching agreement on all the issues of divorce. If the mediator is a lawyer, he or she may draft the separation agreement for review by the couple's separate attorneys; or, the mediator may simply prepare a memorandum of understanding that is used by the lawyers as a guide to prepare the separation agreement. After the agreement is signed, a complaint for divorce is filed in the court so that a simple uncontested divorce can be obtained.

Client-Negotiated Settlement

Some clients may negotiate their agreement without the help of a mediator. Then they either draft the agreement themselves or have one of their lawyers draft it. After the agreement has been signed, one of the lawyers files for divorce, and a simple uncontested divorce is obtained.

WHICH APPROACH IS BEST FOR YOUR CLIENT?

The four options described above can be seen as four points on a continuum. At the one extreme is the lawyer-centered litigated divorce, in which the role of the lawyers is primary and the venue for the process is the court. At the other extreme is the client-negotiated divorce, in which reliance on professionals—especially lawyers—is minimal and the couple does everything themselves but file the papers. It is even possible for the clients to draft their own agreement and to file all documents themselves—but for most people this is not a practical option, because the filing details are too complicated.

Almost all couples should choose option 2 or option 3. Very few people are able to negotiate their own settlement without any professional help. If there are no children, if support is not an issue, and if the assets are simple, then this might be a realistic option. But for people with children and the normal complications of setting up two households, it is unlikely that they will be able to negotiate these complex details without help. There are too many places in which the unresolved agendas of the marriage can derail the discussion and produce suspicion, misunderstanding, and deadlock.

Option 1, the lawyer-dominated litigated divorce, should be used only when one or both spouses cannot move forward without a fight. Only when one spouse is threatening unreasonable action or is engaged in dangerous behavior is the protection of the court needed. And the only advantage of filing for divorce early and before a settlement is negotiated is to secure the protection of the court. So, if a parent is threatening to take the children and run or is denying the other parent access to the children, refusing to pay support, or seizing the assets, is it necessary to secure the jurisdiction of the court at this early juncture. And if it is a case of domestic violence or one that involves child abuse, the jurisdiction of the court is necessary to protect the victims. But the use of this option probably applies to less than 10% of all cases.

For the roughly 90% or more of clients who should not begin by filing a divorce complaint, the choice is between a collaborative-style lawyer-centered divorce and a mediated divorce. In the collaborative lawyer scenario, the lawyers still take a central role in developing and negotiating the settlement. Although this is superior because it eliminates the expense and coercion of litigation, it still pushes the clients to the periphery, because they tend to communicate through the lawyers and assume a passive role in the negotiation. This means that the process does not strengthen communication between the clients and the client does not assume full responsibility for the details of the settlement.

This brings us to mediation, which I believe is the best choice for most of the divorcing population. Most couples are capable of succeeding in mediation, and when they do, the results promote long-term adaptation. In mediation the mediator makes it possible for the couple to have discussions that they probably cannot have themselves. The mediator establishes the agenda, brings technical knowledge to the table, and monitors the dialogue to suppress hostile and self-defeating comments by either party. Mediation has the best chance of producing an agreement to which people are committed, because they themselves have shaped it. One of the most dramatic indicators of the success of mediation is that very few mediated settlements lead to postjudgment litigation. In contrast, if we look at lawyer-negotiated divorce settlements, we know that about half will end up back in court within 2 years of the divorce, with people fighting over money and children. This suggests a much higher rate of satisfaction with mediated outcomes and a greater commitment to honoring the agreement. Finally, mediation puts a conflict resolution procedure in place; so, if a couple has a disagreement they cannot resolve after the divorce, they come back to mediation rather than going to court.

The cases in which mediation might not work and in which a lawyer-dominated divorce might be preferable are those that involve a client who is simply too passive to speak for him- or herself and who would be unable to handle the negotiation even with the support of a mediator. Sometimes one spouse is so dominant and the other so submissive that the parties will be unable to negotiate effectively to a fair result. But I regard these cases in the minority and believe that mediation is the first choice for most couples.

ENCOURAGING CLIENTS TO CHOOSE MEDIATION

Because so many clients associate divorce with lawyers and trials and believe that divorce invariably involves a legal battle, it is important for you to learn how to dispel these misconceptions and present mediation as a viable alternative. To this end, I would like to address common myths people have about the role of lawyers and the legal system.

• *Myth 1: Getting an aggressive lawyer will help you win.* This macho myth about being tough leads to nothing but grief. "You have to be tough or you get rolled over." "If I start out tough, she will know that she can't take advantage of me." "She has to know that if she messes with me she'll have nothing left when it's over." These are but a few of the postures I have heard innumerable times. Inevitably, the people who say these dumb things go looking for the toughest lawyer in town. "I want the meanest lawyer I can find. I want a guy who has blood running off his bicuspids. I want the guy who can wipe the floor with her lawyer." And they will find him. And they will end up with a rotten divorce, monster legal bills, and a dysfunctional family.

The truth is that all lawyers are socialized by their training to have aggression in their repertoires. So, when one hires a lawyer with a swaggering aggressive manner, all one assures is that the lawyer will evoke a similarly aggressive response in the spouse's lawyer. So, what is gained? First, the two lawyers will have a difficult time cooperating; so, we can expect much pretrial motion practice. That means they will go to court frequently to seek relief from the judge. They will go to court over temporary support, temporary custody, visitation, control over property, and arguments about discovery. Aggression begets aggression, which begets more aggression. Aggression defeats cooperation, which is what clients need if the divorce is not going to consume them. Every time the two lawyers fail to agree and every time they have to go to court, it will cost each spouse from $2,000 to $5,000. And each time they go to court, the two spouses will be further alienated from each other. Taking a dispute to court does not represent success; it represents professional failure.

• *Myth 2: Be the first to strike.* Many people and too many lawyers believe that by striking the first blow in court they win a strategic advantage. So, they counsel that the client hire a private detective to try to catch his wife cheating. Or they tell the client to close the wife's credit card accounts and drain the bank accounts before she can get to the bank to do the same to him. Or they propose that the client be the first to file a complaint for divorce in court in order to bring the case under the jurisdiction of the court. But the sad truth is that there is no such advantage. The client may even succeed in re-creating his own little Pearl Harbor, but whatever initial advantage may be won will be eroded by the war of attrition that inevitably follows.

So, advise your clients not to strike. Instead, they should stroke. The strategy should be to reassure the spouse that he or she wants to divorce cooperatively. Let the spouse know that there is no intention to file anything in court until the two of them first negotiate a cooperative agreement. Let her know that the client will not cut off credit cards or move money and that he hopes she will do the same. The creation and management of a cooperative divorce is up to each spouse, and it is not something for which either should count on his or her lawyer. Each must model for the other that he or she will not abuse whatever power he or she has, and this provides the greatest chance that the other does not abuse power either. Trust is built over time but destroyed in a minute. Either lawyer, if out of control, can quickly destroy whatever trust exists between the spouses.

- *Myth 3: The Court will offer protection.* Many people think that judges are wise Solomonic figures dispensing justice from the bench. They believe that judges are godlike people who will ferret out the truth, reward the virtuous, and smite the wicked. In truth, the quality of judges varies widely, with the average hovering around mediocre. And judges do not necessarily regard being a divorce judge as a particularly desirable assignment. A judge I knew was being rotated from the divorce court back to the criminal court from which he had been transferred 2 years before. When announcing his new assignment, he said, "I am so happy. I'm going back to rape and murder and things I understand."

Judges are either appointed or, in some states, elected. Judges who are appointed have to pass muster with legislative committees and have to be politically acceptable to the party in power. So, political considerations play an important part in the appointment of judges. Judges who have to be elected are about as competent as any other people who run for local political positions. The judge who hears a case may or may not have much experience in family law. The rotation system operating in many jurisdictions moves judges around from one area of the law to another without regard to whether that judge has much expertise in that particular specialty. The judge who hears your client's case may have specialized in criminal law and know nothing about divorce, families, or psychology.

So, from a quality assurance perspective, it is best not to be too optimistic that the client will get a judge with the expertise, sensitivity, intellectual horsepower, or wisdom necessary to do justice to the case. And even though your client can appeal to a higher court if he or she does not think the judge's decision is fair, such appeals are expensive, time-consuming, and difficult to win. And even if one prevails on appeal, appellate courts simply remand the case back to the original judge for rehearing. Judges are human and don't like it when their decisions are successfully appealed.

Judges are also very busy. They do not have much time for any single case, because they are under considerable pressure to keep their calendars moving. Much of their review of documents is done by their law clerks, who are usually recent law school graduates. So, the person who may be most significant in deciding your client's case may be a 25-year-old who just graduated from law school and who has almost no experience in family law or in life itself. Because judges are so busy, they often do not take the time necessary to fully understand complex legal matters. Some shoot from the hip, and when they make mistakes the client has to live with them or face the expense of an appeal. So, one only submits to this very imperfect system when there is absolutely no other choice. Your clients are better off staying as far away from the judicial system as they can.

- *Myth 4: "I am better off letting my lawyer talk for me."* Because the legal system seems so complicated, many people are afraid that if they speak for themselves they might make some damaging admission or say something that can "be used against them" in some unknown way. So, to be safe, they decide that they ought to just let their lawyer do the talking for them. Unless the client is particularly naive, gullible, or passive, I think that this is a bad idea. In truth, divorce law is not all that complicated, and when it is there is usually a lot of wealth involved. For most middle-class people, there is little in the way of complicated legal doctrine that will affect their divorces. Most of the problems faced by divorcing people are practical problems, not legal problems. How do we stretch the income that barely supported one household so that it will support two households? How do we help the kids adapt to changed circumstances and still be OK? These are the real problems of divorce, and they are solved by reasoned practical deliberation. The more talking done directly by the couple, the more efficiently they will solve the problems. The more their lawyers are interjected, the more complicated becomes the communication. In the end, the clients must make the decisions that will shape their lives. Trying to do this through the lawyers is like trying to thread a needle wearing ski mittens. Each client is the world's foremost expert on his or her own life, and the lawyer is not even a close second. The lawyer is there to give legal advice. She (or he) can tell her client what she *thinks* might happen in court. She can tell what she *thinks* the law says about the situation. But she is no better than your client in understanding or communicating with your client's spouse.

Communicating through lawyers is a tricky proposition, because the opportunity for misunderstanding is so great. Clients often end up paying many thousands of dollars in unnecessary legal fees just because the lawyers happen to dislike each other. The divorce bar in most cities is a rather small group, and the lawyers who specialize in divorce tend to know each other. Some like each other, and others despise each other. Bad blood between lawyers makes for extra litigation, because there is no trust and no goodwill; so, each lawyer relies more on formal court procedures to protect him- or herself against the perceived duplicity of the other.

The level of litigation is also influenced by the personality and professional style of each lawyer and how the two lawyers happen to interact. Some lawyers are blustery, while others are quiet and polite. Some are good listeners, while others are not. Some negotiate effectively and win the trust and cooperation of others, while some are obnoxious negotiators and squander one opportunity for cooperation after another. Some lawyers have more faith in the judicial system than others and like to go to trial, while others have less faith in the judicial system and prefer to settle. Finally, some lawyers are just greedy. The lawyer argues that he (or she) cannot do an effective job unless he first conducts exhaustive discovery, obtains every possible relevant document, and takes the deposition of every conceivable witness. A great deal of discovery conducted by lawyers, at great expense, is actually of little or marginal importance. The lawyer takes the position that if one must to go to trial it is important to uncover every detail. The same lawyer also believes that he gets the best deal by holding out to the last minute and then negotiating a settlement on the courtroom steps. There are no data to suggest that such lawyers get a better deal for their clients in the end. But there are plenty of data to suggest that such lawyers generate very large fees.

The serendipitous combination of lawyers' personalities and styles affects emotional costs as well as legal costs. The story of Stan and Julie presented in Chapter 6 is a case in point. When Stan's lawyer counsels him to drain the checking and savings account and Stan follows that advice, the message received by Julie is that Stan cannot be trusted. When Stan's lawyer tells Julie's lawyer that she doesn't think that Stan should pay any alimony, she knows in advance that ultimately Stan will indeed have to pay alimony. She takes this position as a bargaining ploy to keep the final alimony figure as low as possible. But what Julie hears is that Stan wants to abandon her. When Stan's lawyer also tells Julie's lawyer that child support ought to be half of what it needs to be, she is engaging in another bargaining ploy. But what Julie hears is that Stan wants to abandon his son as well. She hears the lawyer's strategic ploys as if they were Stan's real intentions and holds Stan responsible for the emotional content of his lawyer's positions. Very few lawyers fully comprehend the psychological impact that these strategic maneuvers have on the other client. It is one thing to use such techniques in commercial or personal injury litigation, where clients will never again have to deal with each other. But in family matters, where we expect the clients to cooperate as parents for the next 15 years, the results are very destructive.

When the client hands over control to the lawyer, these are the risks assumed. Clients are often surprised by the intensity of the spouse's anger and dismay because they have delegated not only control of the strategic negotiation but also management of the emotions of the case to their lawyers.

PROPOSING MEDIATION AS AN ALTERNATIVE TO LITIGATION

The right approach to control of one's own divorce begins with introducing the concept of mediation to clients. If you are a marriage or family counselor, you will likely present the concept to both parties, either simultaneously or individually. Ideally, both trust you and are willing to follow your suggestion. However, you can suggest mediation even if only one member of the couple is receptive. And if you are an individual therapist who has worked with only one party, you can still recommend mediation and make concrete suggestions to increase the chances that mediation will occur. You need to coach your client on how to recruit his or her spouse to a mediated divorce. It does not matter whether your client is the initiator or the noninitiator. Your client can convince the other spouse to try mediation if the approach is made correctly.

Explain to your client that a good divorce requires collaboration to resolve economic, child-related, and practical issues. And when there are children involved, it will require continued collaboration to raise the kids to maturity. So, it may seem paradoxical that the key to separating well is a complicated task that can only be performed together.

The negotiation of an agreement is a joint task. Even though each spouse is focused on ending the marriage and developing separate lives, both must undertake this joint task, and there is no way around it. Even if they perform this task through lawyers, ultimately the couple will have to reach agreement about how to manage the children, how to manage the income, and how to divide the property. The only question is whether they will choose an efficient way or an inefficient way.

It is important to clarify that negotiation does not mean each will act as if they only have joint goals. We will discuss this at greater length in the next chapter. But it does mean that they will recognize that they have many goals in common and that the ability of each to thrive will be largely determined by how well the other thrives. Because mutual trust may be low, your client must be patient when he or she first proposes mediation. The proposal must be cast in terms of joint willingness to negotiate a cooperative agreement. The proposal should not be made with respect to any particular arrangement. For example, it would not be good to propose that the spouse agree in advance to some particular custody arrangement as the price of cooperation. Here are the elements of the proposal.

1. "*We both seek a decent divorce.*" This is the basic proposition. It casts the divorce as something requiring both parties to act in concert.

> "I have been thinking about the divorce and how we should go about it. I think it is important that we both do it decently, and I hope that you feel the same way. I am aware how easily some couples get into litigation and spend years torturing each other before a settlement is worked out. I think it would be a shame if that happened to us."

2. *Fair results.* The reference to fairness is important, and there should be no specific settlement terms proposed at this juncture.

> "The divorce will be a difficult transition for all of us and especially for the children. We need an agreement that allows the children to retain solid relationships with each of us. We need to divide our resources so that two households can thrive. I want you to know that I am committed to working with you to accomplish a fair and equitable division of income and property. I am also committed to doing it in a way that allows both of us all the time we need to figure this out."

3. *"We should use mediation."* Introducing mediation must be accompanied by information about what it is. Your client should have books, articles, and websites available so the spouse can learn more. It might help to have the names of several mediators on hand. This shows thorough research and makes the suggestion concrete.

> "I have been doing some reading and believe that we should use a mediator to help us negotiate our agreement. A good mediator can help us identify options that we might not think of and can help us to keep talking when we get stuck. I hope you will join me in finding the right mediator for us."

4. *"We should use lawyers carefully."* A common error is to insist that neither spouse consult lawyers out of fear that the lawyers will make a mess. But if your client's spouse is frightened or regards your client as having a negotiation advantage, the insistence on proceeding without lawyers may frighten him or her away from mediation. There is every reason to consult with lawyers but to choose lawyers who will support clients in mediation rather than take control of the negotiations.

> "I am not asking you to do this without the help of a lawyer. I am asking that each of us use lawyers to advise us when we need advice but that we not ask them to take over and speak for us. We each should be free to obtain all the advice we need to do this well, whether that advice comes from lawyers, accountants, or psychologists."

5. *"We both need to commit to not walking out."* A commitment to staying in negotiation even when there are serious disagreements is important for getting past the rough spots. And in my experience, the commitment not to cut off communication is very important to either party as reassurance that he or she is safe. In that spirit, it could be helpful to offer something along these lines:

> "I am proposing that we make a mutual commitment to keep talking until we resolve all issues and that neither of us use the threat to quit when we are frustrated. I promise to stay with it until both of us are satisfied that the agreement works."

Encourage your client to allow the spouse ample time to research and digest this new concept and to become comfortable with it. Pressuring the spouse into accepting mediation will be counterproductive.

HELPING CLIENTS TO CHOOSE MEDIATORS AND LAWYERS

As a therapist you should get to know the lawyers and mediators in your area. Helping clients to choose the right lawyers and mediators can save them untold grief. But it will take some diligence on your part to check out the professionals in town. Their public reputations are not generally a very good guide. For example, in every town there are a few lawyers who enjoy reputations as the "toughest lawyers in town." They tend to have big practices, are seen regularly in court, and tend to dominate local practice. They also tend to be poor choices, particularly for the majority of people who do not seek litigated divorces. You will need to get to know half a dozen lawyers and check their approaches to divorce. Most lawyers are eager to find new referral sources and will be happy to make your acquaintance. It is equally important to be personally acquainted with mediators before referring your clients. A competent mediator can spell the difference between a good divorce and a bad divorce. The spirit of cooperation between the couple and the positive impact on the family dynamic and family finances can redound for years to come. Conversely, an incompetent mediator can botch the process and drive the couple into the waiting arms of litigiously oriented lawyers. Researching and meeting with mediators, therefore, is essential. And, like lawyers, these mediators will be only too happy to have a new referral source.

Initial Considerations in Choosing a Mediator

The old adage "Many are called but few are chosen" might have been written about mediators. For several reasons there are too many ill-trained, inexperienced, and incompetent people representing themselves as mediators, and it will take some diligent effort to find the right mediator. It is certainly possible to find good mediators, but they must be searched out. Over the years, mediation has attracted thousands of practitioners. Because mediation is multidisciplinary, it is not limited to lawyers or therapists. Even if it were, that would not be of much help. There are many people who have earned significant sums of money offering "training" seminars to would-be mediators. When the field was getting under way 25 years ago, there were almost no clients, and very few professionals had any experience as mediators. So, training was a hit-or-miss affair. Most training opportunities were offered as 5-day-long seminars during which participants role-played mediation. Although such seminars can familiarize people with some aspects of mediation, they hardly qualify as "training," because real training involves hands-on learning of a craft. Who would want to consult a physician who had never treated a real patient or a therapist who had never worked with a real client? Yet hundreds, if not thousands, of people with no more training than these programs are representing themselves as mediators.

One would have hoped that, over the years, the education of mediators would have matured with the field and that clinical training would have become the norm. But that has not happened. So many people wanted to be "certified" as mediators and so many mediators sought training profits that the field became stuck and never evolved as it should have. To make matters worse, many state court systems, eager to offer mediation, set up programs that claimed to train and certify mediators. For example, in North Carolina, where I practice, the state supreme court set up a program in which people are certified as mediators by the court after taking a 5-day seminar and observing a "certified" mediator interacting with clients in at least two cases; so, in that state you can be certified as a mediator by the court even though you have never mediated a single case.

Because of the poor job this relatively new profession has done in establishing credible training and certification requirements, neither therapists nor their clients can rely exclusively on the formal credentials touted by mediators. Claims of "certification" and the completion of formal "training" programs are, for the most part, meaningless. This does not mean that one can't find a good mediator. It just means that one can't rely on the formal credentials. What one wants to find is someone who has a great deal of experience and comes highly recommended by other people, including therapists who have referred clients to this person before, lawyers who have represented clients who have been through mediation with this mediator, and where possible, the former clients themselves. Therapists who have successfully referred to mediators for a long time are a reliable source of referrals. One can also use the Internet to review the résumés of local mediators.

As a therapist, you need to develop a list of mediators to whom you can refer your clients, just as you need to develop a list of lawyers who can represent your clients without doing damage. You are looking for experienced mediators. I think that 50 completed cases would be the minimum number a mediator would need to qualify. It takes that much experience to really begin to develop the craft. Avoid mediators who have little experience or who have a narrow scope of professional experience. This is one field in which gray hair (or no hair) may be an asset.

Experience is the most important but not the only criterion. One thing that is not important is the gender of the mediator. I have never believed that men or women are necessarily biased in the direction of their own gender. If all else works, gender makes no difference. So, in the event that the wife insists on a female mediator because she believes that a woman would be more sympathetic to her, a husband can readily agree without fear. And the reverse is also true. If the resistant spouse will be more likely to agree to mediation if the mediator is of the same gender, there is nothing lost or compromised for the other spouse in complying.

Another important issue is whether or not it is important for the mediator to be a lawyer. This has been a subject of considerable controversy over the years. About 40% of mediators are lawyers. Another 40–45% are mental health professionals of one persuasion or another. The rest are from such other fields as accounting, financial planning, and education. Although I do not believe that the profession of origin of the mediator is important in itself, I do believe that the knowledge and skills of the mediator are very important. A divorce mediator needs basic knowledge about divorce law, family finances, family dynamics, and the psychology of divorce. I have met psychologists, lawyers, and other professionals who by virtue of their experience and study are knowledgeable in all these things and quite able to do a creditable job of mediation. I have also met lawyers and accountants who are totally unversed in matters of psychology and family dynamics, just as I have met psychologists who are completely lost when it comes to the technical side of divorce. Anyone who is deficient in any of these areas is not fit to mediate divorces. Sidebar 7.1 summarizes the qualities of a competent mediator.

Occasionally a situation may demand the specific skills and expertise of a mediator with a particular background or credentials. For example, in a case characterized by financial complexity, the probability of finding a psychologist with the requisite knowledge is very low. But most divorces are not very complicated from an economic perspective and do not require terribly sophisticated financial expertise. Ultimately, each client has to analyze his or her own divorce and seek a me-

Sidebar 7.1. Qualities of a Good Mediator

- Expertise in divorce law and economics.
- Expertise in family dynamics and the psychology of divorce.
- Knowledge about the financial aspects of divorce, such as taxes and budgeting.
- Strong counseling skills.
- A reassuring and commanding presence.
- At least 50 completed mediations.
- References from other professionals who have been involved in cases conducted by this mediator.
- References from satisfied individuals who have successfully used the services of the mediator.

diator who has the background and skills most germane to his or her problems.

The Process of Choosing a Mediator

Interviewing and choosing the mediator should be a joint activity on the part of both spouses. It is worth the time and money to interview two or three to get a good sense of what the mediator knows and how the parties relate to this person. The rapport they establish individually will be all-important. Is the mediator a calming presence? Does she seem to know what she is talking about? Is his communication clear and concise? In the end, both parties have to be comfortable. Since collectively they are about to design some very important long-term plans, finding the right person is well worth the extra effort. Both parties should be prepared to pay for such consultants. Professionals who give free samples are too hungry and probably not very experienced. Sidebar 7.2 contains a list of questions to ask prospective mediators.

Styles of Mediation

Because mediation is a craft and depends so much on what the practitioner brings to it, mediators vary in the way they mediate.[1] As in sev-

[1]See Folberg, J., Milne, A. L., & Salem, P. (Eds.). (2004). *Divorce and family mediation: Models, techniques, and applications*. New York: Guilford Press.

Sidebar 7.2. Questions to Ask a Prospective Mediator

Ideally, these are questions you should ask mediators to whom you refer clients so that you can best match your clients and their individual circumstances to the mediator. You should also give this list of questions to your clients, in case they decide to find a mediator on their own.

- Do you identify with a particular style of mediation?
- Under what conditions will you offer your opinion about what the clients should do?
- How many divorces have you mediated?
- Have you studied family dynamics, especially as they apply to divorce?
- Are you knowledgeable about financial matters involved in divorce?
- For complex financial situations, such as clients who own their own business, how will you approach valuation and audit issues?
- Do you have accountants and appraisers you recommend, or do you simply rely on the parties' lawyers or on their own ability to locate these professionals? How much technical experience do you have in coordinating the work of these and other neutral experts who participate in the divorce?
- For unusual cases (such as complex financial situations, unusual religious situations, special-needs children, and the like), how many similar cases have you mediated?
- Do you have references? (You are looking especially for references to lawyers who have represented clients of this particular mediator or therapists who have worked with this mediator.)

eral other aspects of this field, the mediator's style has been the subject of controversy. For example, some mediators will occasionally see each spouse alone. Other mediators have been taught that such "caucuses" are undesirable practice. Some mediators are more dominant and directive than others. They are more likely to make suggestions, provide active leadership, and suggest options and possible solutions when you are stuck. Other mediators are less directive and more facilitative. They tend to wait until the parties have worked out the main issues, and tend to intervene less frequently and in a less obvious manner. Part of the difference is personal style, and part of the difference may be strategy. However, some mediators have developed a notion of "pure" mediation, in which the mediator may only facilitate and never even offer an opinion. Such a mediator ideology is based on the premise of absolute self-determination for clients, in which any mediator intervention that introduces the mediator's perspective is regarded as wrong. I find this approach too rigid. Anything that helps clients reach fair and mutual agreements should be used by good mediators. Those who are trained to be passive in therapy and sit by while the client struggles for insight often do not make good mediators, because they are too reluctant to intervene when needed. From my experience, therapists who are trained in behavioral or cognitive therapies do better than therapists trained strictly in psychoanalytic traditions. Passivity on the part of the mediator is not helpful.

I think clients do best with a mediator who has significant expertise about what works and what doesn't work in divorce and who is willing to share that knowledge. The mediator should be prepared to do anything that the two clients request to help them reach a settlement. What I enjoy most about this work is that it allows me to bring to bear almost everything I have ever learned about anything. Whatever knowledge I have is at the service of my clients, and the creative possibilities are unlimited. The mediator needs to have a vision of what good divorce looks like and some sense of a map about how to get there.

Choosing and Managing Lawyers

Lawyers are useful tools in the same way that my chain saw is a useful tool. Managed safely, my chain saw cuts down a tree; managed poorly, my chain saw cuts off my leg. And so it is with lawyers. I want to help you to empower your clients to manage their lawyers well.

Doing so begins with hiring a lawyer who will support and further your client's central goal—to have a good divorce. Finding a lawyer who fits this description requires research and diligence. The reputation of divorce lawyers can be misleading. The lawyer with the biggest practice or the lawyer who gets the most publicity in your community is not necessarily the best choice. The lawyer who is often in the news for handling controversial cases in court is most likely a lawyer who is too eager to litigate and insensitive to the delicate interaction between the needs of his client and the needs of his client's family. So, the lawyer reputed to be the toughest lawyer in town is probably not the best choice unless one wants prolonged litigation.

This is a point that cannot be stressed enough, especially since it will appear counterintuitive to most of your clients who, possibly goaded by well-intentioned but misguided friends and family, are seeking tough, high-profile lawyers. It helps to have a roster of lawyers you can recommend, as you have of mediators. Your clients will be more likely to make the leap from their preconceived notions if you can speak authoritatively about a particular lawyer's professionalism, competence, and success in serving the needs of his or her divorcing clients. Here are 10 things to consider when you are getting to know lawyers whom you might recommend to your clients. You might also suggest that your clients bear the same consideration in mind when they interview prospective lawyers who might be suggested by others. Sidebar 7.3 contains a list of questions to ask prospective lawyers.

1. *Knowledge of the law and at least 10 years of experience.* To do divorce work well, a lawyer needs some seasoning. She (or he) needs knowledge not only of the law and legal procedures but also of the norms that prevail in the local legal community. She also needs some life experience. If a lawyer has children, it is a plus when it comes time to talk about parenting issues. It is also helpful if she has had some experience coping with everyday economic issues. Clients should not hesitate to ask the lawyer about herself. The client is going to be relying on the judgment and wisdom of this person and needs to know something about her style, personality, and values.

2. *Small law firm.* Divorce is not like corporate law and does not require the complexity of a big law firm. Most divorce lawyers work in firms of 10 lawyers or less. Many large firms have hired one or two divorce specialists to handle the divorce work generated by corporate clients. In my experience, the fees of big firm divorce lawyers are much larger than the fees of lawyers in small law firms. Lawyers in big firms are under pressure to accumulate large numbers of billable hours. They tend to hand off as much work as they can to their associates and bill for the associates' time as well as their own. They also bill for the time of paralegals and secretaries, and every time a lawyer talks to another lawyer or a paralegal or secretary the client gets billed for both. I recently saw a case in which a sole practitioner had represented the husband and a partner in a major firm had represented the wife. Both lawyers had similar backgrounds and experience. The husband's legal fee was $23,000, but the wife's legal fee was $85,000 for the same case.

3. *A calm, reasoned, and pragmatic approach that assumes your client's case is going to settle.* One does not want an excitable lawyer, and one

Sidebar 7.3. Questions to Ask a Prospective Lawyer

Satisfactory answers to these questions do not guarantee that your client will end up hiring a good lawyer, but they may help weed out the bad ones.

- What are your fees?
- How much is your retainer?
- Do you demand a retainer if a couple is in mediation? (A client in mediation should not need to pay a retainer.)
- How extensive is the discovery that you usually conduct? (Some lawyers are so compulsive and obsessive that they won't leave a singe stone unturned even if there is little gain in the activity. They may spend $10,000 of their client's money chasing $1,000 in supposedly hidden assets. Clients must seek a lawyer who takes the long view and comprehends the interests of both spouses.)
- How many divorce cases do you take to trial in any given year? (A divorce lawyer who actually goes to trial more than three or four times a year should be avoided.)
- What percentage of your cases are settled in any given year? (A divorce lawyer who settles less than 95% should be avoided.)
- How many of your cases settle before any court action has begun? (A lawyer should litigate only as a last resort.)
- How long does it take you to settle a case?
- Are you committed to making sure that your client is on speaking terms with his or her spouse when the divorce is completed?
- Do you have children? What is your role in their lives?
- What is your caseload? How much time do you have to devote to each case? How long does it take you to return phone calls?
- What is your attitude toward divorce mediation? Have you represented clients who were in mediation? Can you supply the names of mediators who worked with your clients?
- Can you supply references from other professionals with whom you have worked? (Lawyers cannot divulge the names of their clients but should be able to give you contact information for other professionals familiar with their practice.)

certainly does not want a lawyer who stokes the client's indignation and anger. What your client should look for is a lawyer who is calming and who counsels a pragmatic problem-solving approach to the divorce. There are lawyers who hook the client in the initial interview by acting as if they are incensed by the injustices that have been visited upon her (or him) and urge her to seek vindication in court, with the implication that he is the right gladiator to get justice for the client. But it is the same lawyer who, after 2 years of litigation, comes out of a conference with the judge just before the trial is to begin and tells the client to be pragmatic and to settle.

4. *An assertive rather than an aggressive personality.* You do not want a bellicose warrior type to represent your client. You want someone who is assertive rather than aggressive. An assertive lawyer supports the client's interests without antagonizing other lawyers. Assertion is rational, but aggression is not. Nobody can be offended by the quiet assertion of a point. But most people are offended when the same point is made with anger and personal animus. Counsel your clients to steer clear of angry lawyers or lawyers who brag about how they win all their fights in court. Instead, encourage your clients to seek a lawyer who seldom *has* to fight in court, because his style helps promote cooperative settlement. When interviewing a prospective lawyer, engage him in discussions about his style of practice and how he sees the world. Is he an optimist or a pessimist? Does he regard other people as essentially decent or does he see the world as full of dangerous, duplicitous people. His way of thinking about people will shape how he counsels your clients and how he relates to others. A suspicious, hostile, or depressed lawyer should be avoided at all costs.

5. *An understanding of the needs of children.* Most people are acculturated to believe that it is intrusive to inquire about the personal life of a prospective professional. In particular, many schools of psychology have emphasized the importance of the therapist as a *tabula rasa,* onto which clients may project their own personal issues and who scrupulously avoid divulging even small details about themselves. Overcoming this predisposition is important if you are to properly screen lawyers for your clients. Do not be afraid to inquire about their family lives—especially how much contact they have with children. If your client has children and might disagree about custody, visitation, or other child-related matters, then it is especially important to discover the lawyer's experience with children in general and his or her own children in par-

ticular. Being a parent can lend a significant dimension to the lawyer's understanding of a couple's parenting issues. Your inquiry into the lawyer's family situation does not have to be inquisitorial or even very formal. Since most people like to talk about their kids, you might be able to engage the lawyer for a few minutes on that subject. If the lawyer is a woman, find out what role her husband plays with the kids. If she is divorced, find out what kind of parenting arrangement exists between her and her spouse. If the lawyer is a man, ask what role he plays in the lives of his children. This will enable you to ascertain the lawyer's viewpoint and determine if he or she is a good match for your client.

6. *A willingness to support clients in mediation.* If your client chooses to pursue mediation, he or she will still need to consult a lawyer from time to time. If, for some reason, the mediation is unsuccessful or is only partially successful, the lawyer's role will expand. Some lawyers are downright antagonistic to mediation, and your clients should avoid working with them. Others are skeptical or ambivalent about mediation, and their support cannot be counted on; they may end up sabotaging the process. The most desirable lawyers are those who wholeheartedly support clients who are trying to mediate successfully. But to locate a lawyer with this attitude, you must learn how to ask the right questions. Does he (or she) believe in mediation, from a philosophical point of view? Does he regard it as a practical alternative? How many of his clients have been successful in mediation? Since mediation has been growing for the past 20 years, an experienced lawyer who has not had numerous clients who have succeeded in mediation probably does not provide real support for the process. There are some lawyers in the communities where I mediate who ruin every case in which they have ever been involved. So, when clients tell me that they are going to use one of those lawyers, I warn them that they are wasting their time in mediation if they continue seeing that particular lawyer. As a therapist you must be willing to provide similar direct guidance regarding lawyers who compromise their clients' attempts to mediate their divorce.

Undermining the success of mediation can often be subtle. For example, some lawyers tell clients that mediation only works when the lawyer is present at each session. As noted in the preceding chapter, this is a decidedly inferior way to conduct mediation. The lawyers invariably want to take over, and the ability of the clients to shape their own settlement quickly gets submerged in the competition between the lawyers. It makes mediation more expensive and more complicated to schedule. So, don't be misled. Real divorce mediation reduces the role of lawyers to that of advisor and consultant and does not have the lawyer acting as surrogate and negotiator. Lawyers who need to be central to every discussion and who have to take over are inconsistent with the objectives of mediation.

Supporting clients through mediation also requires the patience to fully explain legal and technical aspects of the case. Some lawyers are not willing to do this. These lawyers will not be appropriate for clients who wish to pursue mediation for several reasons. One is that mediation places control in the hands of the client and demands that the client be proactive and oriented toward independent judgment. Lawyers who are threatened by a client's need for understanding are accustomed to having passive clients who trust their knowledge and judgment. Other lawyers relish the control they wield by withholding supposedly technical information. But if your client is reasonably intelligent, there are no legal concepts too complicated to understand, so long as someone is willing to explain them. Since this is the primary reason to retain an advisory lawyer while the mediation process is under way, it is important to make sure the lawyer can do this with grace and patience. If the lawyer is condescending or impatient, or if he or she makes everything sound mysterious and complicated, keep looking.

7. *Someone who does not counsel dirty tactics.* It almost goes without saying that lawyers who counsel dirty tactics should be altogether avoided. The dirty tricks I am concerned with involve acts that begin the divorce on a note of bad faith. We have talked about raids on the bank accounts and safe deposit box as classic dirty tricks. Some lawyers will support a man who wants to use the threat of a custody fight to beat his wife into submission on economic issues. A divorce that begins with threats or unilateral grabbing of assets almost always goes sour. And lawyers who encourage or even support such tactics are to be avoided if your client wishes to have a good divorce.

Although your clients should not retain these lawyers, you should still file their names in your rolodex. Under certain circumstances, you might even recommend that your client consult one of these "dirty players." Once a husband or wife has professionally consulted a lawyer, the lawyer is now "conflicted out." This means that he or she cannot represent the other spouse. Residents of small cities are often advised to consult all the most predatory, litigious lawyers in town. Although it can be costly, it means that none of these undesirable lawyers can represent the opposing spouse. This is especially helpful if the spouse is hostile and unlikely to be amenable to mediation.

8. *Someone whose fees are reasonable.* You can't get something for nothing. All divorce lawyers bill for their time, and the more successful the lawyer, the more he or she can charge. Most divorce lawyers have had many clients run up large bills that they could not or would not pay. Consequently, many lawyers want to get a substantial retainer, a payment in advance against which they can bill. Their retainer agreements usually provide that when the retainer runs out the client either must stay current or must make another payment in advance. If a lawyer thinks a case will take a lot of time he or she is usually looking for a large retainer. I have seen initial retainers as high as $25,000. But most lawyers will seek about 15–20 hours of payment in advance.

How much your client will end up paying depends on several factors. One is the demand placed on the lawyer's time. An insecure client in need of daily reassurance or clarification from the lawyer can run up an enormous bill as the daily phone calls add up. Many lawyers bill for every phone call and most will charge one-sixth of an hour as a minimum charge. So, if the lawyer charges $300 per hour, every phone call costs $50. By the end of a long case, the phone calls can amount to several thousand dollars. Clients should be encouraged to turn to their therapists rather than their lawyers for emotional reassurance and handholding. A divorcing couple should also be encouraged to negotiate as much as possible between themselves, thereby minimizing the need for lawyers and enabling them to keep legal bills down.

As you screen potential lawyers for your clients—or as you advise your clients who wish to find their own lawyers—you should ascertain their hourly rate and then compare it to the hourly rate of other lawyers in your area. Your client should be prepared to pay average rates but should be wary of lawyers who have the highest rates in town. But hourly rate is not the only important factor. It also matters how many hours the lawyer spends on each task and how much discovery the lawyer proposes to do on any given case. Several lawyers I know insist on seeing every check that the husband and wife have written during the past 5 years. That might be justified if the case were really going to trial, but to do that in every case just adds many unnecessary billable hours to the bill. And if a client's case necessitates discovery, the lawyer should be required to seek the client's permission before demanding depositions, expert reports, or the filing of a motion in the court. This enables your client to exercise at least some control over costs. Although most divorce lawyers are not accustomed to such accountability, it is completely commonplace in the corporate and commercial world.

Lastly, I am unaware of any data showing a positive correlation between the size of the legal fee and the quality of the results obtained for the client. Generally, the more the parties spend on legal fees, the more contact they have had with the courts, the angrier the divorce, and the worse the result. There is no absolute winning in divorce court, only different degrees of losing. Every dollar spent on legal fees constitutes the measure of the couple's failure to manage their divorce well.

9. *The gender of the lawyer does not matter.* As with mediators, the gender of the lawyer does not affect his or her ability to represent your client. It is not unusual to hear people assume that if you are a man you should hire a male lawyer and if you are a woman you should hire a woman. Such an assumption is based on the premise that men are biased toward other men and women biased toward other women. However, over 25 years in the business, I have seen nothing that justifies such an assumption. Every skill that makes a good lawyer is equally distributed between men and women. And every character deficit and vice that makes someone a lousy lawyer is also equally distributed. I have met decent, competent, and humane male and female lawyers. And I have met stupid, insensitive, and cruel lawyers among both men and women. So, when you find a lawyer who you think can do a good job, has a winning personality, the time for the case, and a reasonable approach to legal fees, keep the person's name on file to recommend to your clients. Whether it is a man or a woman is genuinely unimportant.

10. *Someone who has time.* Some lawyers who are just starting out may have a lot of time on their hands because they have no clients. And other lawyers may have too many clients and not enough time. Nothing is worse than having a lawyer who does not have time to give you what you need when you need it. Most very busy lawyers hire associates to do much of the work for them. In a well-managed practice, lawyers don't take on more than they can handle. But many practices are poorly managed, and many lawyers take on more than they can do well. These are the lawyers who take a week to respond to a client's call or to a call from the opposing lawyer. They are the lawyers who file court documents at the last moment or are forever seeking delays and adjournments because they have not had time to get to any but the most urgent tasks. At a minimum, this is the lawyer who will drag a case out forever and only complete it when the court deadlines make it absolutely neces-

sary. Your clients should not use a lawyer who does not have enough time to handle his or her cases efficiently and quickly. In litigation, delay begets delay and extends the time you and your family have to live in limbo.

If your client's ego or insecurity demands a "star" lawyer, in time this may become problematic. If the star lawyer is a good manager, your client will find him- or herself pawned off on an associate who is supposedly being supervised by the lawyer. The associate may have less experience than the star lawyer. And even though the associate's time is billed at a lower rate than that of the more high-profile and experienced partner originally hired, your client gets billed double every time the two lawyers talk to each other. On the other hand, if the star lawyer is poor at time management, lacks organizational skills, and tries to do too much, your client will not receive the attention he or she needs.

CONCLUSION

Laypeople tend to exaggerate the importance of lawyers' reputations. Generally, I have found that the lawyers with the "big" reputations have simply done the best job at self-promotion and have played to the myths that people need hard-nosed, tough-guy types who will beat up on the other guy (and supposedly get the best result). But, for our purposes, the lawyer most likely to help produce a good divorce does not fit that profile. There are some divorce lawyers who are competent professionals who can do a good job in court when necessary but who would prefer to help the client avoid that process. These lawyers are gentle people, have decent values, and have some sense of the psychological ramifications of their legal maneuvers. For the most part, they do not have "big" reputations. So, here again, the therapist can be the voice of common sense and encourage the client to find a lawyer who can do the job without unnecessary hostility or litigation. That may not be the lawyer to which the client is intuitively attracted, and it definitely is *not* the lawyer whom the client's friends and family are encouraging the client to hire.

8 Supporting Clients through Settlement Negotiations

Once the decision to divorce and its ensuing crisis and the separation have been achieved, the third–and ultimately the most important–stage is the negotiation of the settlement agreement. It is here that the divorcing spouses design the financial and parental blueprint for their futures. It is also here that there exists a large opportunity for the therapist to play an important role in helping clients manage their negotiation successfully.

As discussed previously, clients can choose several ways to negotiate. They can let the lawyers do it, either in or out of litigation; they can try to do it themselves without professional help; or they can negotiate with the help of a mediator. In this chapter I will be assuming that they are working with a mediator or–less desirable–negotiating themselves. My comments about negotiation will apply only indirectly to the lawyer-dominated negotiation, because clients play such a small role in that process. My comments also apply whether the therapist is seeing the couple or only one partner.

If we assume there is a mediator, then what role is left for the therapist? Once again, the role is that of a coach. Your job is to help your client manage the process without getting in his or her own way–to continually help the client distinguish between feelings and long-term interests and analyze the emotional consequences of legal choices. If you understand more about the negotiation process, you are better able to help the client identify negotiation strategies that advance rather than retard the cause of peaceful divorce. You are not there to duplicate the job of mediator. Instead, you are there to help the client manage his or her feelings as they arise and bear on the negotiation process.

DIVORCE NEGOTIATIONS AS UNIQUE

Many clients have had experience in business negotiations and may even regard themselves as accomplished negotiators. But many of the assumptions they bring with them may not work well in divorce negotiations.

In a business context, the negotiators do not have an intimate connection with each other. The deal is focused on money and on finding a mutually profitable solution. In the negotiations that accompany litigation on contract matters or in personal injury litigation, there is minimal prior contact and no anticipated future contact. The focus is on the deal, not on the relationship. Divorce settlement negotiations are different, because there is a powerful history of a relationship. If the couple has children, there is also the certainty of a long future relationship. Even after children are grown, there will be future contact at weddings, events related to grandchildren, and other family events. And if the children are younger, the relationship will be more involved, requiring weekly contact and coordination. So, the focus in divorce negotiations cannot be exclusively on the deal, because the shape of the deal will have great consequences for the continuing relationship between the spouses, and how that relationship evolves will influence the ways they can build satisfying new lives.

Regrets about a negotiated deal differ considerably between business and divorce scenarios. If one side thinks he didn't get a good deal following a business negotiation, he will have regrets but limited recourse. If there is an ongoing business relationship, it may be strained by the "buyer's remorse" of one of the parties, but it will not affect the core of his life. It's just the opposite in divorce. If the parties negotiate a deal that one of them regards as unfair, the dissatisfaction will reverberate through both of their lives. The husband's resentment about paying too much support will color how he relates to his ex-wife and even to his children. Her resentment about his paying inadequate support will affect her willingness to cooperate with him on other issues. Such feelings reduce the inclination to accommodate the other when he or she seeks help. If she feels that she did not get enough support, she will retaliate through the kids, who will show up at his house begging for a new pair of sneakers because "Mommy doesn't get enough child support to be able to buy us shoes." A residual sense of unfairness will invariably sour the ongoing relationship and affect the children.

Divorce settlement negotiations cannot focus only on the deal but must also have an eye focused on how the deal will affect the relationship in the future. This means that it may sometimes pay to make concessions that one might otherwise not have to make. The husband's lawyer may advise him, for example, that the child support guidelines require him to pay $100 a week even though the budget the two partners have worked out suggests $150 a week. The husband can stand on his rights and refuse to pay any more than he has to. Or, he can focus on his long-term interests and pay more. Standing on one's rights is often not helpful when the result is inconsistent with one's needs and interests. Knowledge of one's legal rights is an important element of information. But standing on one's rights has much less utility than many people think; and one needs to understand the high transaction costs of limiting what one does to "the letter of the law." The emotional costs are often not worth it, and this is an area of decision making in which lawyers are often not very useful. It is an area in which therapists can be most helpful.

The negotiation is also an opportunity for the couple to create the model for how they will interact in the future. If they are going to be raising children together, the negotiation is a mutual opportunity to develop the protocols necessary to living in peace. It is their opportunity to establish a cordial yet businesslike approach to solving problems and resolving the inevitable disputes that will arise in the future. The measure of health of any relationship is its capacity to manage conflict. In the negotiation of the settlement they will establish the precedents that will shape the conflict resolution capacity of their future relationship. So, if each one limits his or her negotiation to grudging concessions shaped by the minimal requirements of their "legal rights," that will be the tone of the relationship going forward. So the tone that they maintain during the negotiation will influence much more than the terms of settlement.

Case Study: Larry and Dana

Larry and Dana are trying to resolve the equitable distribution issues of their divorce. The issue at the moment is that when the couple bought their house 15 years ago Dana used $40,000 from her inheritance as the down payment. The house has appreciated a good deal, and the couple has paid off most of the original mortgage; so, there is about $200,000 in equity. Larry believes that they should split the equity in the house 50/50 between them. But Dana believes that she should receive the $40,000 back plus interest before they divide the rest:

> "That was my inheritance. I will never get one again. When your mother dies, you will receive an inheritance that you will keep for yourself. Why should you walk off with half of my inheritance? I'm not going to give into your bullying, and I am not going to let you get away with being selfish once again. If I have to fight for this, I intend to do it. My lawyer says that the judge will give this back to me before dividing what's left, and I intend to have it whether you like it or not."

Larry does not see it that way at all:

> "For 15 years I supported this house. I made the mortgage payments. I renovated the kitchen, landscaped the yard, and built the deck. When the house needed painting, I did it, and when repairs were needed I used my free time to make them. I poured my sweat into this house. And while I was busting my butt working on the house, you were out playing tennis or shopping or wasting your time with your friends. Even considering your contribution to the down payment, I contributed much more than you. I don't see how it's fair for you to get more than half after all these years. I know you don't give a damn about fairness, but you are not going to get your way on this one. I spoke to my lawyer about this, and he told me that because you commingled your inheritance with the house it is no longer exempt property and any judge will give me half. I am not accepting less than half."

COMMENTARY: Larry and Dana are off to a bad start here. They have different perspectives about how the contributions of each during the marriage should be reflected in the distribution of the equity of the house. But, instead of each asserting his or her interest in a respectful manner, each is wrapping the statement of the problem in gratuitous personal attacks, thus creating unnecessary resistance.

DIVORCE NEGOTIATION AS PARADOX

One paradox of divorce negotiation is that each party often demands of the other the very behavior that was missing in the marriage; had it been there, there would not have been a divorce in the first place. "Damn it. You have been acting like an adolescent for 20 years. Now you're going to have to grow up!" Larry and Dana are caught up in a symbolic replay of one of the struggles that was at the heart of their marital discord. They were never quite able to work out how much each would contribute to the marriage, and each always felt that the other was holding back and not doing his or her fair share. Dana was resentful that Larry never acknowledged the contribution her family had made to their material comfort, and Larry had always resented the amount of time that Dana spent pursuing her hobbies and interests.

The second paradox of divorce negotiation is that it requires one to behave reasonably when one doesn't feel reasonable. People feel angry, distrustful, betrayed, indignant, and even bitter. And if their behavior and demeanor in negotiation reflect their feelings, negotiation will fail. Such feelings shape recriminations, personal attacks, sarcasm, ridicule, and stonewalling. All of these behaviors will repel the other and bring the negotiation to a halt. They will also convince the spouse that the partner wants to injure him or her and seek revenge and that the partner is a hopeless candidate for a cooperative parenting arrangement. So, the only viable alternative is to refrain from acting out one's feelings during the negotiation. Here is a vital role for the therapist, who is paid to listen while the client expresses strong feelings and prepares to negotiate calmly and without intense affect.

Agreement versus Contract

There is more than a semantic difference between an agreement and a contract. Lawyers negotiate contracts–formal signed exchanges of promises enforceable in court if necessary. But if all the divorcing couple negotiates is a contract, they will not have accomplished enough. In my experience, at least half of all couples who negotiate through lawyers and sign contracts are back in court within 2 years fighting over children and support payments. A return to court not only is expensive but also contributes to the steady deterioration of the relationship. It is really a testament to the failure of the negotiating effort. In law school we were taught that a contract requires a "meeting of the minds." That is, both parties have to have a mutual understanding of the terms of exchange. But a meeting of the minds does not necessarily mean that either party regards the contract as just or even workable. Contracts are often crafted out of grudging last-minute concessions made to avoid a fight or a trial. Contracts do not necessarily mean that either party is committed to the deal or that either party will honor it in spirit as well as legal detail.

Where people are committed to the deal, I speak of genuine agreement rather than mere contract. If the couple is really in agreement, it means that both will abide by the terms voluntarily because they regard the agreement as fair. It does little good to go to court to enforce a contract. I have seen innumerable people get worn out trying to enforce a separation agreement when a recalcitrant ex-spouse refuses to comply over and over. In truth, a spouse who is hell-bent on sabotaging the agreement can get away with it because courts are reluctant to really punish those who default. Contracts cannot perform. Only people can perform. When a couple is divorced, they need to be able to rely on good-faith performance from each other and not rely on the courts. However we define a good divorce, a divorce in which people repeatedly go back to court is a bad divorce by any definition.

An agreement is not just a meeting of the minds; it is also a meeting of the hearts. The partners may still feel angry at each other when it is over, and both may be relieved to be divorced. But if they have a genuine agreement, they can get on with their lives in a way that they cannot if the two of them are still tearing at each other. It is for this reason that I urge clients to know their rights but to approach them with caution.

Behavior, Not Feelings

A client must be coached to cooperate with a spouse whom she may resent and toward whom she feels distrust and even dislike. But how does one cooperate with someone toward whom one has such negative feelings? Throughout this book, I urge the therapist to encourage the client to focus on behavior rather than feelings. Feelings should be expressed in therapy, not to the spouse. There is little to gain and much to lose by using the negotiation to vindicate one's feelings. "You were the cause of this divorce, so you have to suffer the consequences, not me!" is a proposition driven by feelings that will do nothing but alienate the negotiating partner. I urge clients to accept this fact: there is no vindication available for the feelings they have within the negotiation room. There is only one measure of the usefulness of each statement made in negotiation: how well does it serve to recruit the cooperation of the other party? If it makes the other less likely to cooperate, it is self-defeating. If it evokes cooperation and trust, it is productive. A statement does not have to be conciliatory to be effective, and I am not suggesting that your client surrender or cave in whenever there is a disagreement. But it is important to express that disagreement in a productive manner.

You may object: "All this is well and good, but what does my client do if the other spouse engages in these self-defeating behaviors?" I will suggest some tactics for managing this problem below. But, for now, understand that one of the most effective ways to shape the behavior of another is to model that behavior for him or her. Unwillingness to counterattack and retaliate will likely defuse the attack. Mediators can be helpful by intervening and correcting the self-defeating behavior. So, when a client says something nasty, demeaning, or blaming to the other, I will stop the attacked spouse from responding and ask the attacker, "Marjorie, help me understand how what you just said and the way you said it will encourage John to work well with you here." And, unless Marjorie is a complete dolt, she gets the picture. I find that it doesn't usually take too long to extinguish such behavior if the attacked spouse follows my cue and doesn't retaliate or defend.

If you are a couple's therapist, you may be able to adopt this approach and may well be using it already in your sessions with your clients. But even if only one party is your client, you can help by role playing negotiations and showing how attacks can be reframed and expressed differently.

COACHING YOUR CLIENT THROUGH NEGOTIATIONS

As your client goes through the process of mediation, there will be inevitable ups and downs. After some sessions she may be optimistic; after others she may be pessimistic. As a therapist you are well positioned to help the client analyze what is happening in the negotiation process and modify his or her behavior when appropriate. Because they are so anxious about the outcome, it is easy for clients to overlook the importance of monitoring their own behavior during the negotiation sessions, and it is also possible for them to misinterpret the behavior of the spouse. Good mediators do a lot of monitoring, but you as therapist are able to help the client go deeper into an analysis of why the negotiation is developing as it is. You can also play an important role in validating feelings and support not provided in mediation. In this next section I will review some of the behaviors that can advance or retard negotiation. If you can help your client understand these and act accordingly, you will provide an invaluable service.

Self-Defeating Behaviors to Avoid

There are five types of behaviors that are almost always self-defeating in divorce negotiations, because they antagonize without accomplishing anything. They often arise from the misconception that you can intimidate a negotiating partner into submission. And even if they are occasionally successful in securing submission, submission is not agreement.

Shaming and Blaming

This involves criticizing the spouse's character and using knowledge of the spouse's history and vulnerability to hurl accusations designed to humiliate. It can be accompanied by name-calling and other forms of put-downs.

> "You are just no damn good! You lied about the affair, and that makes you a no-good liar. And you are so greedy that I don't know how you can even show your face around here."

Attacks on the character and personality of the spouse underscore the attacker's unreliability as a negotiating partner, evoke defensiveness, invite counterattack, and frighten the spouse into litigation.

> "You never did your share, because you were too lazy and selfish to bother."

This is totally counterproductive. It rehashes the most contentious issues of the marriage and creates such a poisonous atmosphere that no further negotiation is possible.

Acting Helpless and Passive

In this scenario, the person effectively denies any responsibility for the divorce, adopts a passive position, and demands that the spouse absorb all the change and dislocation.

> "I didn't want this divorce. If you want it so much, *you* leave."

Threatening and Intimidating

Here, the bullying is designed to change the other person's mind.

> "Take it or leave it. But if you don't take it, I will fight you until you have nothing left."

In my experience observing thousands of mediations, threats almost always harden the negotiating partner's resistance and completely undermine the credibility of the person issuing the threats.

Cutting Off Communication

Threatening to discontinue direct negotiation kills the chance of a cooperative divorce and bespeaks a client's lack of negotiating skill more than it does objectionable behavior from the spouse.

> "I'm sick of your whining and bitching. From now on, let the lawyers do the talking."

All of these statements are understandable in that they reflect feelings of hurt, anger, and frustration. It is difficult for your client to sit on those feelings when he or she believes he or she is being unfairly provoked.

The role of the therapist here continues to be one of helping clients choose to not act out in ways that damage the negotiation process. I often suggest to my client that "you are not a trout, and you do not have to rise to the bait." Clients can be taught to choose not to respond to criticism and attacks. "What you are saying about me is interesting and I shall reflect on it. Now, can we get back to what's relevant?" Even though we reflexively want to defend ourselves when we feel attacked, the choice not to respond kills the attack far more effectively than do denials and counterattacks. With the therapist validating the client's feelings and coaching the client when to duck, negotiations will continue uninterrupted.

Behaviors That Help Negotiation Succeed

Just as there are behaviors and approaches that will invariably spell the end of successful negotiation, there are others that can promote a successful outcome.

Inviting the Spouse to Negotiate through Mediation

Your client's spouse may take the lead and invite your client to negotiate a settlement. If he or she does so, the client will, we hope, be gracious and accept. The client will also express his (or her) appreciation that she has invited him to negotiate and that she wants to shape an amicable settlement. He will take the opportunity to tell her that he shares her desire for a fair and amicable resolution and that he wishes her well. If she has not invited him, then he needs to invite her. I use the term "invite" purposely here. When we invite someone, we assume some responsibility for that person's comfort. We take the initiative to create the contact and implicitly express at least the spirit of solidarity. That is the spirit that we are trying to create. An invitation acknowledges the person's right to decline but expresses a hope that he or she will accept. It is an optimistic beginning.

If the spouse is skeptical, your client should not try to talk her out of her skepticism. Rather, he should acknowledge it and the fears that go with it. He should use the invitation as an opportunity to reassure and to express his own determination to arrive at a mutually acceptable and workable resolution. Respecting the spouse's skepticism is probably the most effective way to dispel it. It is less threatening for the skeptic if he or she is reassured that the commitment is only for 1 hour at a time and that the two parties will mutually decide at the end of the first session if they want to schedule a second.

It is helpful if your client has researched available mediators in advance of the invitation to mediate. If the two spouses have discussed mediation previously, they may already have a mediator in mind. If not, you should inquire among the professionals you know to get a few names of mediators for them to consider. If your client's spouse is not familiar with the concept, mediation books, articles, and websites should be provided.

Engaging in Active Listening

There is nothing like marital deadlock to induce despair. Each spouse desperately wants to be heard and understood, and each thinks that everything the other has to say has already been said before. So, they interrupt each other, try to talk over each other, and before long the attempt to communicate shuts down. It is for this reason that so many people think that they will never be able to negotiate with their spouse. It is also this pattern that requires a mediator to make it possible for the two spouses to talk to and understand each other. The mediator will serve as the communications traffic cop and direct traffic to avoid a collision. Clients should be coached to follow the mediator's lead.

But even with the help of the mediator, clients will not be heard if they do not follow some simple procedures. These may appear counterintuitive at first, but, once learned, they are very effective. Here is what I explain to my clients. As a therapist, you can explain this to your clients as well.

- You will be heard and understood only in proportion to the extent that you listen and understand. In other words, the key to being heard is listening.
- "Listening" does not mean simply biding your time while you wait for your chance to talk.
- Listening does not mean simply observing silence as the spouse talks while using the time to plan in your head what you are going to say next.
- Listening means paying attention not only to what is being said (content) but also how it is said (the message). This is active listening.

Active listening has two components. The first is listening to the content of the message.

> "I don't think it's good for the children to stay overnight with you on school nights."

The second is listening to the emotional message and noting the affect with which the message is delivered.

> "When the children are away, I worry about them and I miss them terribly."

If this is delivered with a worried expression, it is important that your client try to understand what feelings accompany the statement. Active listening means taking steps to assure the other person that both the message and its emotional content have been heard.

I tell my clients that the easiest way to convey understanding is a simple summary of what they have heard and what they think matters most to the spouse.

> "So, as I understand it, you are worried that if the children stay overnight with me they will not get their homework done, and you will miss them and be lonely. Do I understand correctly?"

If your client has missed something, the spouse will correct the misunderstanding. But when this is done, the spouse will know that she has been heard and understood. This leads to two outcomes. First, because she knows that she has been heard and understood, she won't feel the need to repeat herself. And second, she is likely to imitate the behavior that your client has modeled. With the help of the mediator and some active listening skills, your client will be able to have a dialogue that has not been possible until now.

Affirming Conciliatory Gestures

In the course of negotiations there will be many issues on which clients disagree, some big and some small. The mediator should set the agenda. As a mediator, I move away from issues on which clients get stuck, seeking agreement on other issues and returning to the hard ones later. In the course of the process, it is likely that each client will make concessions to each other. She may change her viewpoint about a parenting issue and agree to the children's spending more time with the husband. He may agree to move to an apartment or to stay close to the children rather than moving closer to his work. Each will make concessions on property issues and support issues.

This approach will be very effective even outside the mediation setting. It is important that your client affirm the spouse whenever he or she agrees to something that has been sought but not previously agreed to. Although they are getting divorced, they are still connected emotionally to each other in many ways, and each continues to desire the approval of the other. It is very discouraging when someone makes a concession in negotiation but gets no acknowledgment for it. Failure to acknowledge conveys the feeling that the other believes that he (or she) is entitled to the concession or that concessions will now be taken for granted. If your client reinforces the concession or conciliatory gesture, it makes the spouse more likely to do it again. If your client acts as if the gesture is a victory for him or a defeat for her, it will reduce the chance of further concessions from her and raise her fear that she is being taken advantage of. This does not mean that every concession has to evoke a counterconcession. But it costs nothing to say "I really appreciate that you have agreed to that because it means so much to me. I am very encouraged by the progress we are making, and I hope you feel that way too." Conciliation begets further conciliation.

Paying Attention to Tone

As relationships deteriorate, people tend to disagree in an increasingly unpleasant manner. They become more and more frustrated with each other, and the frustration is reflected in the tone of voice that they use when talking to each other. Tone, independent of the words used, can convey not just frustration but also anger, plaintiveness, contempt, and ridicule. So, two things may be happening. First, each may become "allergic" to the tone of the other.

> "When she starts that whining, I just lose it."
>
> "When he starts using that angry condescending tone of his, it just totally turns me off."

So, tone can independently derail what would have otherwise been a completely reasonable message. By tone alone, we can make others feel intimidated, demeaned, and put down. None of those feelings will induce cooperation or enable each to hear the legitimate needs of the other. If this has been a problem, there are several ways for clients to monitor their own tone of voice. First, they lose nothing by acknowledging that their tone may, on occasion, be offensive.

> "Sometimes I get carried away because I'm frustrated, and I know it's wrong. Please tell me when it happens so I can fix it."

The client can also request that the mediator cue him or her if he or she thinks that the tone is becoming a problem.

Refusing to Take the Bait

Divorce engenders fear, and people who are afraid often act in ways that are unpleasant and offensive. So, what happens if your client follows my advice, moderates her (or his) tone, listens carefully, and tries to understand her spouse's needs, and while she is doing this her spouse continually acts aggressively and obnoxious? Is your client supposed to just take it without striking back? The answer is yes.

The client needs to be reminded that he (or she) does not have to defend himself against every attack or criticism. He cannot be harmed by words. Part of what is going on may be related to routines of attack and counterattack that evolve as if they were following a script. She attacks him for being insensitive; he attacks her for being picky. They may have developed a complex choreography of mutual accusations and put-downs as if rehearsing for a performance on stage. So, her attack cues his counterattack. Her indictment evokes his defense of "not guilty." But why bother responding to unproductive provocation? The mediator is not a judge, and your client does not have to convince the mediator that he is being maligned. His angry defense to her attack just makes the mediator's job more difficult. Most mediators do what they do because they get professional satisfaction from helping people reach agreement. Mediators do not like personal attacks and are generally more concerned with the tone and behavior than they are with the content of the message. The client need not worry that the mediator will turn against him. His calm demeanor and his refusal to be drawn into unproductive verbal sparring will actually win the mediator's sympathy for him. Don't attack. And when attacked don't defend. In time the other spouse will get the message. I am aware that some of what I advise here may run counter to the impulse of the therapist to get the client to stand up to verbal abuse and refuse to be put down or diminished by the spouse. But this is a time to focus on successful negotiation. The marriage may well be ending because one spouse talks to the other in an abusive tone. But the time to fix that has passed. Refusing the bait is not submission to abuse. It is simply a refusal to be distracted by obnoxious behavior.

Acknowledging Convergent Interests

One of the problems with adversarial relations is that they tend to focus us on areas of disagreement rather than areas of agreement. Divorcing couples have many interests in common, and it is helpful if they spend some time in negotiation identifying convergent interests. Certainly, an obvious area of convergent interests is the welfare of the children. Although there may be some disagreements about how the interests of the children can be best achieved, the common objective is worth reiterating. The couple also has parallel interests. Each has an interest in building a new life, and it is in each of their interests that the children obtain the permission of each to like the new partners each chooses in the future. It is in the interest of each that the other thrives, because their children will thrive only if both parents do. The review of convergent interests is a good exercise whenever the two parties get stuck on some issue, because it maintains perspective and reduces the gloom that arises when they momentarily despair of ever reaching a comprehensive agreement.

So, encourage your client to focus on minimizing differences instead of exaggerating them. She is demanding $1,000 a week in child support, while he believes that $800 is more than enough. It is true that they are $200 apart in their views. But it is also true that they are 80% in agreement and that their positions are much closer than they are disparate. So, the thing to say is: "Look, we are only $200 apart. What can we do to compromise on that so that we both end up with something closer to what we believe is right. If I was able to stretch to $900, do you think that you could live with that?" I have often had couples come to see me after they have been engaged in litigation for years. When I explore with each of them what they need to resolve the matter, I discover that they are within 5% of each other's positions but are unaware that they are so close. Because the communication between lawyers and between lawyers and their clients is so inefficient, couples may live in limbo for months or even years when they are, in fact, within easy reach of a settlement. The adversarial culture is a pessimistic culture. It is easy to become riveted on differences and miss the degree of real underlying agreement. So, encourage clients to frame their positions in terms of convergence rather than divergence: "I have heard your viewpoint and think that we are very close and believe we could reach agreement with relatively minor modifications" is much better than "I don't care what you say–I am not going to budge a dollar over $800 a week."

Thinking Future, Not Past

I touched on this point in the preceding chapter, but it is important enough to reiterate here, because it is one of the most common roadblocks to successful negotiation between divorcing couples. When I teach mediation techniques to professionals, one of the strategic interventions I urge on them is to keep the couple focused on the future and not the past. I routinely tell couples that in over 3,000 cases I have never succeeded in helping a couple reconcile their conflicting versions of their past history together. Perhaps, if I had unlimited time, unlimited polygraphs, and the ability to assemble witnesses, I might be able to get a couple to come to common agreement on the history of their marriage. But, even if I had these unlimited resources, what would be the point? People have different versions of their history because they have had such different experiences. Your client has lived the past 20 years with her husband, and he has lived with her. They have had radically different experiences and have come away from that experience with very different beliefs about what happened and what it meant. Not only is it a waste of time to wrangle over what happened or who was wrong, but also it is destructive, because it just generates more pessimism.

Most arguments about marital history have two themes. First is the struggle over who was right and who was wrong. The parties seldom agree about this. But there also is the inevitable attempt to link the other's wrong behavior to the proposed distribution of resources.

> "You were so neglectful of the marriage that you don't deserve half the assets. While you sat on your ass and did nothing, I

was busting mine to earn us a good living. Because you did so much less, you should get less."

"It's outrageous that you even think such a thing. I did everything for this family. All you did was go to work and then come home and expect to be served like a king. Don't tell me that I deserve less than you did."

History almost always is a reprise of blame, vindication, and just desserts. It is a waste of time and energy in divorce negotiations, and although I would hope the mediator would intervene and refocus the discussion on the future, it is much better to avoid the endeavor altogether. Although the therapist may still have work to do with the client to help the client understand the past, supporting the client in mediation requires a continual focus on the future.

The couple's past may be troubled and irreconcilable, but their future is quite different. The different ways the two experienced the same events contaminates the past but not the future. It is much easier to decide what will happen in the future than it is to decide what happened in the past. Historical references by each only trigger defensiveness and resistance. So, statements about history, particularly ones that attempt to justify why one should get more, are inflammatory but not productive. As soon as one spouse hears it coming, her resistance rises, and instead of working on solving problems she is preparing to defend against an attack. The easiest way to defuse such comments about history is to say:

"I can understand that you may feel strongly about that, but I don't believe it will help us reach agreement if I respond. So, I am going to respect your thoughts about that, but I am not going to try to talk to you about it."

This is a respectful response that acknowledges her but declines to engage in a discussion that can't lead anywhere useful.

Planning and Preparing

Good negotiation requires planning and preparation. Although neither spouse can predict everything the other will do or say, each can be prepared to provide needed information and can think through many of the likely scenarios.

The first task is to prepare the necessary information. Each issue requires its own preparation. If the two need to negotiate about parenting schedules, they can each prepare a proposed schedule showing where the children would be each night over a 2-week period. Even though they may not be in agreement, the schedule helps focus on the areas of agreement and disagreement and facilitates discussion. When they get to financial issues, preparation is vital. The information they will need is outlined in Sidebar 8.1.

If this package is assembled early, the parties will not have to interrupt discussions because they do not know the value of some asset. The mediator will be grateful, because it allows him to move them or her along without unnecessary delays. Obtaining information is a collaborative venture. It does not matter who gets together the information but only that the parties have it when they need it.

The second aspect of planning is a strategic analysis of the issues. Each party needs to think through how the problems of both spouses might be solved. Clients should be coached to look at problems from their spouse's perspective as well as their own. An issue is resolved only when both regard the solution as workable and fair; so, trying to see the issue from the other's perspective is as important as seeing it from one's own. If, for example, they anticipate that they disagree about how long the wife can stay in the house, each can prepare cash flow analyses showing each possible housing scenario. This will provide a concrete

---

Sidebar 8.1. Information to Prepare for the Financial Negotiation Process

- Three years of tax returns.
- All current statements for bank accounts, brokerage accounts, and retirement accounts.
- Any appraisal of real estate.
- A completed statement of assets and liabilities.
- If there is a defined benefits pension plan, obtain a copy of the plan document.
- Current statement showing all debt including mortgage, home equity loan, credit card accounts, or other debt.
- A completed budget.

---

and nonspeculative basis to hash out the issue. Written budgets and proposals move things along more efficiently than just verbal descriptions.

Using Neutral Language

We have already discussed the use of neutral language in the preceding chapter, but it is so critical that I would like to briefly recap.

- Monitor the choice of words, avoiding insults, put-downs, sarcasm, negativism, condemnation, name-calling, guilt, and blame.
- Use "I" statements instead of "you" statements.
- Validate the other person's point of view–for example, "I understand you want to see the children more often, but I also want time with them."
- Don't counterattack. Instead, try to disarm the attack–for example, "I understand you are upset, but when you call me names, it makes it hard for me to agree with you" conveys information but limits the affect attached to the message.

CONCLUSION

Negotiating the agreement is the final act that the couple must do together. But the purpose of the agreement is to draw up a plan for separate lives in the future. The greatest danger to effective negotiation is the tendency of people to want to vindicate their feelings and hurts from the past in a document that attends to the future. It cannot be done, and the sooner clients figure this out, the faster will be their ability to negotiate a fair and workable agreement. If the client's impulse to vindicate the past is his or her own worst enemy, then the therapist is the client's best ally. By continually refocusing clients on their long-term interests, helping them to distinguish subjective feelings from their true interests, and helping them understand the costs of acting out their feelings, the therapist can help keep the client on a path to successful negotiation. Sidebar 8.2 presents a brief summary of how the therapist can best support clients in their divorce negotiations.

Sidebar 8.2. The Therapist's Role in Supporting Clients through Negotiation

- Managing clients' emotions.
- Validating feelings.
- Providing emotional support.
- Focusing on behaviors required during the negotiation process rather than feelings
- Helping clients focus on future goals instead of past history.
- Helping clients focus on desired goals (cooperative agreement) rather than "legal rights" and vindication.
- Coaching clients in the dos and don'ts of negotiation strategy.

Dos

- Invite the spouse to engage in mediation.
- Engage in active listening.
- Affirm conciliatory gestures.
- Pay attention to one's tone.
- Avoid taking the bait.
- Acknowledge convergent interests.
- Use neutral language.
- Do your due diligence–plan and prepare for the negotiation.

Don'ts

- Don't counterattack.
- Don't shame or blame.
- Don't act helpless or passive.
- Don't threaten or intimidate.
- Don't engage in personal attacks.
- Don't cut off communication.

9 Custody and Parenting

Custody is the one area of divorce with which therapists have long felt comfortable. Lawyers acknowledge that therapists are the experts in this field, and the judicial system routinely recruits therapists as expert witnesses to help the court decide which parent should get custody or whether some proposed visitation scheme would be in the "best interests of the child." Numerous books have been written to guide the therapist through the process of custody evaluations and preparation of testimony. I will not, therefore, devote any energy to repeating what already exists elsewhere in great detail.[1] Notwithstanding their appeal as drama, however, custody fights actually occur in relatively few divorces. Rather than tell you how to participate in custody fights, I will focus on helping you avoid them by educating your clients. I believe that most of the custody battles that do occur are the result of client ignorance coupled with lawyer error and can be averted by early and effective intervention on the part of a therapist.

Most of the harm done to children in divorce is not the result of custody fights. Rather, children are harmed by the continuing high level of conflict between their parents. This conflict may center on child-related issues such as visitation or may be related to economic issues.[2] If the therapist provides firm leadership by educating parents about how their own behavior affects the children, all but the most disturbed of parents will be influenced. So, in this chapter I want to present you with an overview not only of the legal aspects of custody but also the impact of the divorce process itself on children. You will learn about the numerous critical choices–emotional and practical, not only

[1]See, for example, Stahl, P. M. (1999). *Complex issues in child custody evaluations*. Thousand Oaks, CA: Sage.

[2]Heatherington, E. M. (2003). *For better or worse: Divorce reconsidered*. New York: Norton.

legal—that must be made by parents, and you will be given the tools to help parents make choices that will be of maximum benefit to their children.

POPULAR IMAGES OF CUSTODY

It is unfortunate that the popular media have made such a mess of the subject of custody. Perhaps the media is pandering to millions of soap opera fans by presenting sensational images of children being torn away from a parent. We have numerous movies, television programs, and bad novels in which one parent struggles to take a child away from the other because of some allegation of bad or unfit parenting. Although such depictions make good drama, they create unnecessary fears in the minds of parents who are about to be divorced. Many clients who come to see me are scared to death that they are about to "lose" their children. Fortunately, it seldom takes long to calm them down, because the realities are very different from the fictional depictions of custody fights.

Custody fights occur in only a small percentage of all divorce cases. Remember that few divorces ever go to trial and that in most of these the key issue is custody of the money, not custody of the kids. However, although there are few actual custody trials, there are many threatened custody fights—and the damage to children is about the same. In the past thousand divorces I have mediated, only one has deteriorated into a custody fight—a trial in which the judge ruled about custody. That is not because I am a magician, but because my mission is to put out rather than stoke the fires of fear.

The truth about custody issues is far different from what most laypeople and many therapists believe. If approached gently and intelligently, the subject of how to parent the children is almost always resolved without a struggle. Most of the issues that arise between divorcing people are based on fear and on honest disagreement that lends itself to enlightened discussion and negotiation.

AN OVERVIEW OF THE LAW OF CUSTODY

I will talk about custody in this section and then not deal with it hereafter in the remainder of the book. Custody has become a poisoned concept. It connotes that one parent "wins" the kids and the other parent "loses" the kids. Custody is, by its very essence, an adversarial concept; so, many states are beginning to substitute the term "parenting" for the term "custody." I applaud the change and have adopted it in my own discussions. Traditionally, custody was awarded to the parent who "won" the divorce. Remember that until 40 years ago almost all divorce was based on fault, and one way that the losing party was punished was by the loss of the children. In many divorces, the loss of custody meant the complete disenfranchisement of the noncustodial parent. The parent who won custody had absolute control over the children and over the access of the other parent to the children. So, 50 years ago, the loss of custody could indeed be a dire event.

In the post-World War II era, modern psychology began to influence the courts to award custody based not on marital fault but on the "best interests of the child." This, coupled with the assumption that women were better connected emotionally to the children, meant that the mother usually was designated as the custodial parent. But the courts also recognized that children needed contact with both parents in order to develop correctly and so usually "awarded" the noncustodial parent, typically the father, visitation rights. If the father lived within a reasonable distance, he was usually "awarded" alternate weekends with the children. Increasingly he was also "awarded" some access during the week and on holidays. So, by the early 1970s, the routine and classic custody arrangement was one in which the mother had custody and the father saw the children every other weekend and on Wednesday nights.

The 1970s brought yet another shift, this time one that favored fathers. As the movement for women's rights and sexual equality gained steam, more fathers began to assert the right to equal treatment and fought against the assumption that the mother's sole custody was indeed the best arrangement for the children. Fathers fought against the sense of disenfranchisement that came with the designation of "noncustodial" parent and bitterly resented their designation as visitors in the lives of their children. A movement for equal treatment was expressed as a demand for either an equal chance of being awarded custody or as a demand for joint custody, in which the children would spend equal time in each household and the parents would have equal decision-making rights and equal access to school and medical records of the children. By the late 1970s, many couples were negotiating joint custody agreements in which the children would typically spend 1 week or 1 month with the mother and then spend 1 week or 1 month with the father. Although this worked well for many couples, it also worked poorly for many others.

JOINT LEGAL CUSTODY

By the 1980s, scholars and judges were looking much more critically at the issue of joint custody, and lawyers started seeking alternatives. The joint custody scenario, with its numerous moves and changes, was often disruptive to children who now had no primary residence. For many families it worked well. But for many couples the achievement of a perfect or mechanical 50/50 division of the children's time was too impractical. Particularly as children grew older, adolescents resisted and sometimes rebelled against the frequent moves, and the joint custody arrangement was seen to not usually work.

The question was how to avoid the sense of disenfranchisement of the noncustodial parent while constructing a parenting system that gave greater continuity to the children. The answer was old wine in new bottles–the concept of joint legal custody, with one parent–typically the mother–designated as parent of primary residence. This concept makes explicit that, by having joint legal custody, the parents will make all the important decisions affecting the health and welfare of the children consensually. Each parent has equal access to school and health records, and each has equal rights to attend meetings and conferences involving the children. And, instead of talking about visitation rights, we talk about parenting schedules that delineate the time the children will spend with each parent.

Joint legal custody, with one parent designated as the parent of primary residence, has become the most common form of parenting in American divorce. Although it often looks similar to the old pattern of having the mother in charge and having the father spend alternate weekends and Wednesday nights with the children, it does provide at least symbolic recognition of the important place the father occupies in the life of the child. And, of course, the specific schedules vary from couple to couple, as we will see in the next section.

BASIC ISSUES IN JOINT CUSTODY: DECISION MAKING AND SCHEDULING

Think about what it involves to be a parent. First, one has to nurture the child by providing basics such as food, clothing, shelter, and love. One also has to teach the child how to get along in the world as well as provide educational opportunities and recreation. In other words, one has to take care of the child so that he or she thrives and develops. So, nurturing also includes making decisions for the child until he or she is able to make them without the parent. The parent decides where he goes to school, who will provide medical care, and what activities are acceptable. We generally distinguish between decision making and nurturing, although the two are really closely related.

When a couple divorces, the parents have to divide the responsibility for raising children in some reasonable and workable manner. They have to decide how they will take care of the child, how decisions will be made, and by whom. If they are unable to decide, the court will decide for them. Usually the court will declare that one of the parents will be in charge and that the other parent will play a secondary role.

The two aspects of the parenting agreement, then, are decision-making protocols and the parenting schedule. When we call the parenting arrangement "joint legal custody," we require the parents to make important decisions consensually. When we call the arrangement "sole custody," we say that the custodial parent has unilateral decision-making authority. The second aspect is the schedule. This specifies where the children will live, what days of the week they will spend with each parent, and with whom they will spend which vacations and holidays.

Both aspects of the parenting agreement–decision making and the parenting schedule–can be subject to fear and dispute between the divorcing parties. It will be important for you as a therapist to recognize and address the fears and concerns that couples typically experience when it comes to decision making as well as parenting arrangements.

Decision Making

As mentioned, joint custody involves joint decision making. That concept can be distressing to many parents, but worries over control of the children are more often symbolic than substantive. It is easy for divorcing parents to become agitated about how they will make important decisions for their children. But, in fact, the importance of such decision making is often overblown, and the therapist has the opportunity to breathe some realism into the discussion. What constitutes an "important decision"? With reasonably normal healthy children, the number of decisions of earth-shaking importance is actually quite small. Is Johnny going to private school or public school? Is Johnny going to get a religious education? Is Johnny going to have an operation to fix his knee? Major decisions such as these come along maybe once or twice a year. And would any reasonable parent expect to make such a decision without at least some consultation with the other? These obviously fall into the category of decisions that should be made jointly. However, most of the decisions that shape a child's life are small and have an impact only cumulatively. Can I stay up late tonight to watch TV? Can I have a new pair of sneakers? Can I get a new video game for Christmas? These decisions are, of necessity, made by the parent on duty without prior consultation with the other, because it is too burdensome to talk about such minor issues.

By refocusing the discussion from the abstract to the concrete, the therapist can take the heat out of the discussion. Ask clients to count the number of important decisions they made for the children in the past year. They will be surprised at how few there actually were. Then ask if they would make such a decision without consulting the other parent. Few will say no. Finally, encourage your client to discuss the difference between major and minor decisions with his or her spouse, if you are not seeing the couple together. I have calmed down innumerable parents with this simple intervention.

Parenting Schedules

In approaching parenting schedules, it helps to frame the discussion in terms of the most important needs of parents and of children. Once these have been clarified, it becomes easier to construct schedules that meet the needs of all family members.

What Parents Need

Each parent needs two things with respect to the kids. First, each needs to spend significant time nurturing the children and enjoying the company of the children. As we raise children, they become integral to our identity as a person in that our role as parent becomes an important part of our sense of self. Any parenting agreement has to attend to the need of each parent to spend time with the children. A second need of each parent, in my experience frequently overlooked by women, is the need for substantial time off from the children. Most people divorce hoping to meet someone new and in time connect with a new mate. Each will be dating and trying to build a relationship with someone new. To do this, each needs time without children. When one is dating, the children are a liability, not an asset. If a divorced person becomes involved with a new potential mate, that person will, at best, tolerate the divorced person's children. He or she will rarely welcome them. So, if a person is only available with his or her kids in tow, few potential girlfriends or boyfriends will stick around for long.

The ability to understand the need for time off from the children often depends on whether one is the initiator or the noninitiator of the divorce. I find that the person who does not want the divorce and has not yet made peace with the fact of divorce has also not yet figured out that he or she will have a life in the future. I can recall several couples in which the noninitiating wife fought every overnight that the husband sought with his kids. She came up with one far-fetched reason after another until he was totally frustrated. Finally I asked her if she had much of a support system in friends and family. She replied that she did not. So, I asked her who provided her with companionship and support, and she answered that it was the kids. Then I asked how she felt when she did not have a child at home, and she answered that she felt devastated and lonely. Only then were we able to talk about other ways to not feel devastated and lonely so that she would not have to clutch the children so hard.

As you help a client to think through his or her need for an emotional life independent of the children, his or her need for time off from them will become apparent. If your client does not yet feel such a need at present, he or she will as time goes on. As the client becomes more engaged in building a new life, the need to hold on to the children all the time usually diminishes.

What Children Need

Children need time with both parents. As we discussed at length in Chapter 2, children need both parents to care for them and love them and for both to be involved, at least to some extent, with their activities.

But what children need most of all is for the two parents to be able to cooperate around issues affecting the children. They need them to cooperate around financial matters so that they don't end up in the middle when the parents disagree about money. They need the parents to be pleasant to each other when they move between households, and they need them to be reasonable with each other in accommodating changing schedules. They need encouragement to be comfortable in both households. And when one of them develops a relationship with a new significant other, they need the permission of the other parent to like the new person.

Most scholars who study divorce agree that the level of cooperation between the parents is the most powerful predictor of how well children will adapt to the divorce. Some data suggest that the level of psychological problems is no greater in children of divorce so long as there is a high level of cooperation between the parents. It does not really matter what the "custody arrangement" is called, or the specific schedule is not that important, so long as each parent gets significant time with the children and the parents have a cooperative arrangement.

GENDER AND FEAR

As divorcing parents begin to explore possible parenting arrangements, they are not always aware of their needs–especially time off from the children. Nor are they necessarily aware of their children's needs. Instead, they may be all too aware of their concerns and fears. As a therapist, it will be important for you to allay these fears, which often differ depending on the gender of the client.

Most families are still organized along traditional gender-based lines, although some families may deviate from this norm. It is true that the majority of mothers are employed at least part-time. But in addition to employment, they also tend to administer the lives of the children. It is mostly mothers who are found in the waiting rooms of pediatricians. It is mostly mothers who are found at parent–teacher conferences, and it is mostly mothers who stay home when a child is sick. It is predominantly mothers who schedule play-dates and extracurricular activities for children, and it is mothers who chauffeur the children to after-school activities. I am not suggesting that there are no fathers in the pediatrician's office, the school conference, or the family car as it takes the kids to soccer practice. There are men in attendance. But it is primarily mothers who perform these functions, not because of any anti-male conspiracy but because both partners want it that way.

So, at the risk of political incorrectness, it is necessary to recognize that in most cases mothers are both practically and emotionally closer to the children than are fathers. That is not to dismiss the critical importance or vitality of the father's role. But there is a difference in the emotional connection between mothers and their children, beginning with pregnancy, and continuing through nursing, babyhood, and the early years. In most families, it is the wife who spends more time with the children, especially when the children are small. I have seen a few two-career couples in which everything has been done equally and both parents have spent equal time with the children, beginning in infancy. In that rare scenario, conflicts are unlikely to arise, because the couple will continue their parenting arrangements into the divorce. But conflicts do arise when there has been an unequal arrangement—when the mother has been the primary parent and the father, possibly out of fear of being shunted aside, demands joint custody with an expanded role during the divorce. Understanding the fears of both fathers and mothers will enable you to address them more effectively in therapy and will help pave the way for parenting agreements that are free of conflict.

The Fears of Fathers

Many fathers approach divorce with the fear that they will be effectively cut out of their child's life. Fathers fear that their wishes and preferences will be ignored, that they will lose the opportunity to share the child's life in any meaningful way, and in many cases they fear being replaced as the father by the wife's next husband. In short, fathers fear losing their place in their children's lives.

How well founded are these fears, and how can we allay them? At first glance, the statistics on fathers are not encouraging. About half of fathers default on their child support payments or pay later and less than they are supposed to.[3] Many fathers drift away from their children, and many fathers spend much less time with their children than they otherwise could. Whether this is because they are not interested

[3]*Almanac of Public Policy*, April 1, 2001.

and committed or whether this is because mothers sabotage the father's relationships can be debated at length. But because the statistics include many couples that had children out of wedlock and at a very young age, they do not provide an accurate picture of middle-class educated couples. Among educated couples, continued and robust engagement by fathers is the norm rather than the exception. Indigent teenage parents suffer from so much disorganization in their lives that it is a minor miracle when they can pull off successful parenting of any kind.

The way to allay the male client's fears is by helping him to assert an active interest in his role as parent and insisting that the parenting agreement he will negotiate with his wife maintain full relationships between the children and both parents. As I will explain below, I suspect that his wife will ultimately be cooperative, because it is in her interest to do so unless the two get involved in a rancorous divorce. But it helps if the husband also approaches the subject with an understanding of why his wife might initially be reluctant to accept the concept of joint custody. Men who are outraged that their wives resist joint custody fail to comprehend that they are proposing a new emotional arrangement with the children. A man who understands his wife's fears and concerns is less likely to act on his anger and more likely to seek cooperative solutions. If the usual gender roles have been operative during the marriage and the father is now seeking an equal parenting role after the divorce, he will need to acknowledge, both to himself and to his wife, that he will have to learn some new tricks with the kids.

The Fears of Mothers

In divorce, mothers have their own fears that must be addressed. There are some men who, outraged that their wives are leaving them, threaten to "take away the children" or to "fight for custody" as a way to dissuade the wife from the divorce, or to frighten her into concessions. In divorce, we are seeking a parenting arrangement in which the parents are each involved in the lives of the children and in which the children are comfortable in both parents' homes. Threats of the loss of children often result in defensive attempts by the mother to minimize contact between the children and the father. The tug-of-war that results is extremely destructive. So, it is important early in the divorce for professionals to actively discourage threats and to encourage both parents to foster contact between the children and the other parent.

It is equally important to reassure women at the beginning of the divorce that no one will challenge their role or try to deem them unfit. Since there are powerful stigmas attached to women who give up their primary parenting role to the father, women may fear that by relinquishing time with the children or by giving up their role as primary caregivers, they will be publicly labeled as defective or "bad mothers" and become social pariahs.

Many women who have been the primary parenting figure in the lives of the children also fear a loss of control. They are used to being the primary rule makers for the children. They are the ones who arrange the daily details of their children's lives and during the marriage were rarely challenged by their husbands. Rules regarding dietary habits, bedtimes, choice of friends, choice of clothing, and when to do homework are more frequently made by the mother. Many women worry that when the children are in the father's home, unsupervised by the mother, the rules they have worked hard to enforce will be undermined. Consequently, some precipitate power struggles with their husbands as they seek to minimize the time the children spend with their fathers and as they seek to enforce their own rules and standards in the father's house. These fears need to be addressed and managed by the therapist.

One of the least-addressed fears of women in divorce is the fear of being overwhelmed by the sheer magnitude of what they are expected to do. They are expected to be the primary caretakers for the children, manage the home without help, make a major economic contribution to their own support and the support of their children, and build a new life–all at the same time. In many cases the woman worries that the husband will spend too little time with the children, not seek too much. In the dialogues that occur between lawyers, the focus is typically on asserting the rights of fathers to more time with their children. Lawyers know how to assert rights. Obligations are another matter. For the mother of children with a disinterested or detached father, there is little relief to be had in the legal system. A father who is content to spend minimal time with his children cannot be compelled to spend more. So, the traditional alternate weekend visitation pattern has the children with the father approximately 4 nights a month. This means that they are with the mother up to 27 nights a month, leaving her too little time to build a life of her own. In the modern two-career family, this is often the greatest fear for women and one poorly served by the adversarial system.

The case below is designed to demonstrate the process of guiding a couple from their decision to separate through reaching a joint parenting arrangement that meets the family's emotional and practical needs. Note that each party's fears and decision making (both "major" and "minor" decisions), as well as living arrangements and parenting schedules, will be addressed.

CASE STUDY: JOHN AND MARIA

John and Maria were divorcing after 15 years of marriage. They had two children–Becky, age 11, and Jeb, age 8. John was a successful CPA, a partner in an accounting firm. He had routinely worked 60 hours a week for many years, and the couple had a nice home and some money in the bank to show for the hard work. Maria was employed as a teacher in the public schools. She had chosen that job in order to be off from school when the kids had vacation. Maria had routinely attended to the children, while John put in long hours and earned the money needed by the family. Maria was earning $30,000 a year, and John was earning $200,000.

The couple had been going through marital struggles for many years and had several unfruitful rounds of marriage counseling. Although both had given up on the relationship, they had been held together for years by inertia and a mutual concern for the children. But when Maria found out that John had a brief affair at a convention he had attended, she was livid. She told John that she wanted a divorce and that she wanted him to leave. John was relieved in some ways that the marriage was finally over but was anxious about the children and about his relationship with them. Like many couples, John and Maria had some initial discussions to feel each other out about what the divorce would look like. Maria told John that she expected to stay in the house with the kids. She would agree that he could see them frequently as long as they continued to live with her.

"That's not good enough," said John.

"I want joint custody. I want the kids to live with me half the time. I'm not going to become some visiting father without any rights. I'm just as good a parent as you, and there is no reason for me to be a second-class parent!"

Maria was incredulous when she heard this.

"Where have you been all these years while I've been doing everything for the children? You are rarely home in time for supper. You almost never supervise their homework. You don't take them on errands, and on weekends you say you need to go unwind and play golf. How do you expect to be an equal parent now when you never have before? Forget about joint custody, because I'm not agreeing to it."

Now John became angry.

"Well, I'm not moving out of this house until you agree to joint custody. I'm not just going to leave my house and my kids and everything I worked so hard for and send you a fat check every month. Until you change your mind, I'm not going anywhere. And if the only way I can get a fair shake with the kids is to sue you for custody, I will do so."

John and Maria settled into an angry state of deadlock. They slept in separate bedrooms and were barely talking. Maria consulted with her friends and was encouraged to hold her ground. She consulted several lawyers, who told her that few judges would order joint custody under the circumstances and that no judge would give John sole custody, considering the history of the family. John also talked to friends and cronies. Several advised him to stick to his guns and fight for his rights because they knew too many men who had gotten screwed by their wives. John sought out a lawyer, who told him that the odds were against him in a custody fight but that he might get joint custody, depending on which judge heard the case.

John and Maria each asked their lawyers how much it would cost to take the case to trial. Well, Maria's lawyer opined, it would depend how sour the other economic issues became. In his experience, if custody were contested, everything else was also contested, and if that happened, the cost to her could approach $100,000. John's lawyer said something similar. As neither was willing to commit to such an enormous expenditure, each just hunkered down to see if the other would give in. So, 6 months passed and nothing happened. The atmosphere became ever more tense at home, and the children became gloomy and depressed.

One day Maria received a call from Becky's guidance counselor at school. The counselor told her that Becky was not doing well in school and that several teachers had noted that she seemed listless and irritable in class. Her grades had fallen, and a child that had been an excellent student was suddenly missing homework assignments and flunking quizzes. The counselor suggested that Maria and John come in for a consultation.

COMMENTARY: John and Maria are similar to many couples I have seen. John fears being cut out as a parent. Maria fears that John is seeking something he does not deserve and something that would not be good for the children. But neither is looking ahead at what the family needs, and neither is attending to what the children need right now. Living with divorcing parents can cause depression in children. But neither parent understands how to break the stalemate that is preventing all four of them from healing and moving forward. They get encouragement from others to fight but are intimidated by the cost. They are not willing to go to court, but they don't know how to resolve the issue.

John and Maria attended the session with the counselor a few days after the phone call. After reviewing the teachers' comments, the counselor asked if anything was going on at home that might explain Becky's sudden poor performance in school. When Maria told her that they were on the verge of divorce but were unable to agree on custody, the counselor suggested a probable connection between their struggles and Becky's problems. She said that she had seen this many times and that Becky's academic problems would likely resolve if her parents could get their own issues resolved. She warned that it was extremely important for John and Maria to figure out how to cooperate as parents very soon, before Becky got into long-term trouble. The counselor suggested that they consider mediation, which she had found effective in other cases. They asked for a referral, and the counselor referred them to me.

John and Maria came to see me about a week later. They both appeared to be pleasant and essentially reasonable people who were caught up in the fears that often dominate a divorce. Although they brought all their economic issues as well as their parenting issues to mediation, I will comment here only on the parenting discussions.

John and Maria each summarized their viewpoints. Maria had always been the primary parenting figure and saw no reason to give up that role now. She said that John's role with the children had always been played within a framework maintained by her. John saw the kids as he came and left the house. He might see them at breakfast, but it was she who was preparing their breakfast. The same applied to dinner when he was home—which he frequently was not, particularly during tax season. Although John often attended the children's sports events, it was based on whether it was convenient for him, and it was assumed that whenever it did not suit his purpose she would be there to take care of the kids.

John agreed that Maria's depiction of history was more or less accurate. But he believed that the divorce meant that many things would have to change. For one thing, he was tired of killing himself at work. Last year one of his partners had a heart attack, and he wasn't going to have that happen to him. And it was precisely because his contact with the kids had been based on the assumption that Maria would cover for him that he would need to take more time off from work to spend with the children. He was not about to become peripheral to their lives.

It was also obvious to him that Maria would have to get a job that paid more money. Maria had an MBA and had earned twice the salary of a teacher before the kids had been born. So, if this happened, Maria would have to work more and would have less time to spend with the kids, time that John would have to cover. That was why he wanted a full joint custody arrangement.

COMMENTARY: Although John and Maria appear to be at loggerheads, they have more interests in common than they realize. At the moment, they are still struggling to hold on to what they have in the marriage. They will solve their problems when they move to organizing their lives for the future and recognizing the role that their parenting plays in their long-term future scenarios.

Addressing John's and Maria's Fears

In my discussions with John and Maria, I began to introduce these ideas. I suggested to John that he needed to validate Maria's claim that she had been the primary source of nurturing for the children. With a little coaching, he finally said to Maria:

"I am sorry that I ever questioned your role as the kids' mother. Of course, you have done most of the work, and you have done a wonderful job helping the children to be successful. I hope you will work with me to work out some arrangement in which I can now have an expanded role. I think they need a full and rich relationship with both of us and I will help you in any way I can."

Maria replied:

"I appreciate how hard you have worked to provide for me and the children, and I know that you have not always had as much time with them as both of us would have wanted. I will work with you to keep you central to their lives."

COMMENTARY: John's statement to Maria helped her to relax and not feel so acutely that her identity and role as mother was being threatened. Only then was she able to stop trying to prove that she had indeed played a primary role. In time she was able to do so. Now Maria could exhibit some grace toward John. This small shift in the way the two of them framed the issue set the stage for a cooperative resolution.

Reducing Conflict over Parenting Schedules and Joint Custody

Once the concept of a shared parenting arrangement is accepted, the clients must begin to focus on the nuts and bolts of what that will look like. A few key concepts help lower the temperature of the debate over schedules.

Alternating Weekends

This is the classical arrangement, with few deviations. The exception occurs in families in which one or both spouses work on weekends–for example, policemen, airline pilots, medical personnel, or shift workers in factories. In these families, every other weekend does not work. But for most couples alternate weekends are the rule, because they accomplish several things. First, they give each parent personal time when the children are off from school and the parent is off from work. Thus, the largest block of available time is shared equally. Of equal importance, weekends are the time that most people date and each parent can count on being free every other weekend to pursue a social life. It is interesting to note that alternate weekends are almost universal even in situations where a judge has awarded sole custody to one parent after a custody fight. Alternate weekends are almost a foregone conclusion in most divorces. John and Maria did not argue about weekends, so we moved on to the more troublesome issue of school nights.

Conflicts over Weeknight Arrangements

Weeknights are usually the subject that causes the most stress in parenting negotiations. John and Marie struggled through this issue.

Maria said:

"It's fine with me if the children spend weekends with you, but I think they should spend school nights with me. They're used to me doing homework with them, and I am afraid that they won't get their homework done or that they won't get enough sleep. I think they should be in their home on school nights. You can come have dinner with them and do homework anytime you want, but they should stay in my house. Besides, the confusion of living in two households and moving back and forth will be too much for them."

To this, John responded with great frustration:

"It's just not good enough for you to tell me that I should have the kids only 4 nights a month. How can you say that you want them to enjoy a rich relationship with me, which must be developed in such a small number of nights? That's ridiculous, and I won't accept it."

COMMENTARY: Maria's objections to overnight stays with John during the week are typical, albeit uninformed and unfortunate. It is important that John not overreact and that he let the mediator do his job of educating Maria. Divorce means that children have two parents in two houses and need to spend time with each parent in each house. It certainly introduces a measure of disorganization, and one might as well acknowledge that. Obviously, it is easier to live in one home than two. But in divorce the choices are limited. Either the children spend significant time in both households and learn to manage some initial disorganization and readjustment, or they spend all their time in one house and in effect lose significant contact with one parent. In the latter case, the loss is too significant.

Maria has raised two questions. First is the issue of who helps the children with homework. When I was a child, my parents expected me to do my homework. If I didn't do it, I caught hell from my teachers and received bad grades. Then my parents would be angry, and life would be unpleasant for a while. But it was my problem and my homework. On occasion, if I was stumped by something, I could ask my father for help and he would help. But I had to take the initiative. There was nothing unusual about my parent's approach, and it was no different than that taken by my friends' parents. Today we seem to live in a much more child-centered world, in which too many parents inject themselves as integral to their children's homework. The result is children who cannot sit down and do their homework without a parent hovering by.

Part of the solution depends on how the couple has handled this in the past. If the mother has been the one who has always done homework with the children without the father's involvement, he will have to ease his way into the role, if he philosophically supports the concept of parental involvement in the children's homework. Certainly fathers can help kids with homework as well as mothers can. If he disagrees with the centrality of a parent in a child's homework, he may want to have a discussion with his wife about letting the children become a little more independent and take responsibility for their own work. Although the kids have been accustomed to having their mother on hand, this does not mean the father is obligated to provide the same sort of assistance. The easiest way to institute any change is to try it as a pilot program. So, here is what John was coached to say:

> "I don't fully agree with you about how much we should be helping the kids with their homework, but I am willing to cooperate. Let's have an experiment for a month. I will help them every other week and you help them the rest of the time, and let's see how it works out."

By framing his proposal as an experiment, John avoids a fight and secures Maria's agreement to try. Over time John may be able to get Maria to relax about the homework issue. But this should not determine whether the children stay overnight with their father during the week.

The second issue raised by Maria is the "bouncing ball" complaint. She assumes that if the kids move between two households that they will literally be bouncing about and therefore be too confused to function. Again, in an ideal world it would not be necessary to move kids back and forth. But in the world of divorce some movement between homes is unavoidable. If the two parents are cooperating, some movement during the week will not hurt. The objective is to have the kids spend sufficient time with each parent to achieve the needs that parents and children have for each other. But we want to do so in such a way as to minimize the transitional periods.

If John were to see the children 2 nights a week and wanted them to sleep over with him on Monday and Wednesday nights, that would be a poor schedule, because it has the children moving back and forth almost every day. But if he seeks to have them on Monday and Tuesday nights, it would reduce the number of moves to a minimum. That is a strategy I often suggest to clients. I recommend extending the weekends from Friday evening through Monday morning, when the father sees them off to school. This increases the amount of time with the father without additional transitions. They are already located at his home for the weekend, so they just stay over another night. I find that this is easy for women to accept, and it is appealing to them because it gives them a bigger block of time off from the children.

If the weekend with the father consists of Friday, Saturday, and Sunday nights, then Monday through Thursday nights remain with the mother. If the children spend every Monday night with their father, it would mean that he has them 5 out of 14 nights. If we were now to add Tuesday nights, he would have them 7 out of every 14 nights, or precisely half the time. But in either case, we connect the weeknights to the weekends so that the children only make two transitions each week. In the first case, what I call a 4/1 schedule, he has them 4 nights one week and 1 night the alternate week. In the second illustration, what I call a 5/2 schedule, he has them 5 nights one week and 2 nights the next week. I have found that either of these schedules reduces confusion to a minimum.

The Issue of Equality

We have been raised to believe that equal and fair are nearly synonymous. Equality is so deeply ingrained in political discourse that we almost automatically assume that if anything is less than equal it is unfair and unjust. I find that, for many men, equality of time with their children becomes the symbolic test of whether they are being treated fairly and often becomes more important than the larger question of what works. For men who seek joint custody in the face of resistance from their wives, the divorce may come down to a choice between the equal joint custody and an arrangement in which the children spend less than half their time with the father but enough time to accomplish his objectives. I submit that the issue may, in the end, prove more symbolic than substantive. Let's return to John and Maria:

When I started working with Maria, I found that she could shift her position on things as long as she was allowed to think about new proposals. I began by proposing to her that it would not work well for the children to spend only every other weekend with John. My first reason was that such a schedule did not give her enough time to herself, time that she needed and deserved. It also did not give John enough time with the children to feel he was fully involved. Finally, it wasn't enough time for the children to fully develop a relationship with their father. What did she think might be done to increase the time with the children and their dad?

"Maybe he can come over during the week, do their homework with them and see them to bed. Then I could go out at least for part of the evening," she replied.

"How will you feel having John in your house several evenings a week after you have separated? Won't you feel a need for more privacy?" I asked. I told her that in my experience people are not comfortable having an ex-spouse in their home, and the ex-spouse soon becomes uncomfortable being in his former home. What was her objective in doing it that way?

"I want to avoid having the children leave their home. If he takes them to his house, then they would have to come home at the end of the evening, and that's too much for them."

"Why do they have to come home?" I queried. "If they are at his house already, why not have them stay over once or twice a week?" She repeated that she was afraid that it would cause too much confusion. We talked a while about the lesser of two evils, and we ended the session.

The next week when she came, she said that she would be willing for the children to spend one overnight during the school week with John, and extra time during vacations. But John objected to this plan.

"That won't do it. If she can't do better, I'm going to fight. I don't want a battle, but I'm not going to be pushed out as the kids' father. Every other weekend and one night a week isn't even close to half time. I want half time." I asked John what was important about half the time. "It's only fair," he said. "Fair means equal."

I asked John what an equal pattern would mean. He said he didn't care as long as the number of nights was the same in each household. I asked them to look at a 2-week schedule. Maria was proposing that the children spend 4 out of 14 nights with John. John was proposing that the children spend 7 out of 14 nights with him. Their disagreement was about 3 nights every 2 weeks, or 1½ nights a week. I described a schedule to them that I have seen work hundreds of times. If we expanded the weekend to include Sunday night, the children would be with John every other Friday through Monday morning. That added 2 nights a month. Now, as Maria had already agreed to 1 night a week, if we made that night Monday, then the children, already at John's house through Monday, would now stay through Tuesday morning. On the off-week for John, he would have them Monday night. Now he would have them five nights out of fourteen, which was only 1 night a week less than the half time he sought. This would also address Maria's concern about moving the children back and forth too frequently. John said that he would think about it, but he was still upset because it wasn't equal. I observed that, by adding Tuesday night, the schedule would become equal, because he would have them 7 nights out of 14. Then I asked John to tell me what time he came home at night and when the children went to bed. " I come home at 6:30, and the kids go to bed at 9:30," he said. "So," I asked, "are you telling me that you are willing to spend $50,000 and make a mess of the divorce over 3 hours a week?"

After thinking about it, John replied that maybe it might work if Maria would let him have the kids more during the summer. I asked Maria if she would consider having the kids at John's another night during the summer and if she could accept the 4/1 schedule I had described. She agreed to the schedule during the school year and agreed that the children would also spend Tuesday nights with John during the summer. The matter of parenting rights was resolved.

COMMENTARY: John didn't get his equal-time arrangement. Is this unfair? Fair is such an abstract concept that it is not very useful when we talk about divorce and children. The more important question is whether the schedule agreed by the couple works for all members of the family. With his 4/1 (in a 2-week period, John would spend 5 of each 14 nights with the children) schedule during the school year and 5/2 (in a 2-week period, John would spend 7 of each 14 nights with the children) schedule during the summer, John has enough time to maintain the full, rich, and robust relationship he seeks with the children. Maria retains, at least in her mind, her primary role but gets enough time off from parenting to build a new life. The children get the time they need with both parents. This family has done about as well as it could. If Maria had been comfortable with an equal schedule, that would have also worked well, but frankly the specific schedule is not that important, so long as it meets the needs of the entire family. The range of possibilities is not unlimited. Four or 5 nights every 2 weeks are enough to maintain each parent's place in the children's lives. If either parent has 6 or 7 or even 8 nights out of 14, that is also workable. I have seen few court battles over this subject that made sense in terms of cost–benefit calculations, or net gains and losses.

Household Rules

Parents—whether married or divorced—do not necessarily agree on household rules. People differ on the many aspects of child rearing, from how to discipline the children, to what to feed them, to when to put them to bed, to what lessons to give them and what risks to allow them to take. Some parents forbid TV viewing; others allow unlimited TV access. Some indulge their children, and some believe the children should live more spartan lives. When children live in separate households, there is an unlimited opportunity for parents to get into conflicts. And as in most of the conflicts arising from divorce, most are not worth fighting in that the transaction cost of the conflict usually exceeds the importance of what the dispute is about. Transaction cost refers to the secondary costs of hurt feelings and accumulated resentments that arise whenever harsh words are spoken or one parent criticizes the other.

John and Maria, like most other couples, struggled with this issue.

John and Maria separated and began to live with the schedule they had negotiated. About 2 months later, I received a call from a distraught Maria. "This isn't working. John is doing stuff with the children that I can't approve of, and either he has to stop or I will fight him in court." I asked her to tell me about the problem.

"Well there is more than one problem. First, John refuses to give Jeb his Ritalin, because he says he doesn't believe in giving such medicine to children if they don't need it. So, on weekends he says he won't give the medicine to Jeb. The doctor never told us to skip weekends, and Jeb comes home too wound up after he has been with John. I also found out that John lets the children stay up past their bedtime—and the kids need sleep."

She paused. "Is there anything else?" I asked.

"Yes, it gets even worse." "John took the kids snowmobiling and didn't have them wear helmets. He also took Jeb for a ride on his motorcycle when he knows that I am deathly afraid of motorcycles. When I told him that was irresponsible, he just told me to quit telling him what to do and that he would decide what was best when the children were with him. And worst of all, I found out that John's new girlfriend spent the night with John when the kids were there, and I absolutely won't tolerate exposing the kids to that immoral behavior."

I suggested that she invoke the mediation clause in their agreement and come in for an appointment with John.

COMMENTARY: It is seldom that a divorced couple agrees on all the rules that should apply when the children are in residence with them. Different parenting styles are especially accentuated when the mother who has been the children's primary caregiver and rule maker must make room for a very different parenting style.

There are a few points that I emphasize. The first—and perhaps the most difficult for many single parents—is to mind their own business when the children are in their former spouse's household. For example, a mother cannot expect her ex-spouse to do everything the same way she does it. It will not happen, and if she pushes too hard it just sours the parenting relationship. Most issues are not worth the struggle. Although it is preferable for the regimens in both households to be similar, children will not be injured if their parents feed them differently or if one parent is more lenient than the other. Children quickly figure out that their parents are different and have different expectations and styles. If the father lets them stay up later than the mother, they might be sleepy once in a while, but it's not going to ruin their lives. The same applies to some of the other issues that seem to preoccupy people. Food faddists and alternative medicine devotees may get worked up about what the child eats or what the doctor prescribes, but it's really not going to shape the child's life in important ways. What will shape the child's life is a perpetual battle between the parents. I advise my clients to bite their tongues until they bleed. I urge clients not to precipitate conflicts unless the life of a child is truly endangered. Stupid and reckless behavior that exposes the child to great risk is worth discussing. For example, it is stupid to let kids ride bikes or to rollerblade without helmets and protective gear. It is not acceptable to violate such principles, and one does not break the rule when one objects to such a thing happening when the child is with the other parent.

How does one assess the issue of transaction costs? How can one determine whether an issue is worth the fight? The most important guide is common sense. There is a difference between an ex doing something one doesn't like with the kids and doing something that by objective standards is dangerous. When in doubt, I advise clients to overlook anything that isn't downright dangerous. But there is also another side. If a mother, for example, asks her ex to abide by some rule or regimen with which he disagrees, when should he comply and when should he refuse? Here is where we return to the concept of transaction cost. Is it worth it to assert his autonomy in each instance? How strongly does he feel? If he does not feel strongly about something, it may be wise to give in. If one party feels more strongly than the other, it's not worth the fight. Sometimes we comply with the wishes of others for no reason other than to please, indulge, or even humor them. It's called "getting along." Men often have exaggerated autonomy needs that cause them to get angry when they think someone is trying to tell them what to do. In my experience, most women have trouble understanding this and think that men are just being unreasonable. But this is not a book about gender behavior; it is a book about how former spouses can live in peace. So, I urge clients to pick their fights carefully. One party tries to change the parenting of the other only when the welfare of the children is genuinely endangered. And one defends one's own parenting only when it's really worth it.

Let's see how some of the issues played out when I saw John and Maria. John and Maria came to their appointment angry. John jumped right in.

"She's always trying to tell me what to do. It was bad enough when we were together. It's intolerable now, and she better learn to mind her own business!"

Maria was equally indignant.

"I'm sick and tired of his insensitive adolescent behavior. This is just what I was worried about, and if John can't be a more responsible parent, I will go to court and reduce the amount of time the kids spend with him."

I asked them both to calm down. I also asked Maria to tell me which of her issues she regarded as the least important and told her that we would take that up first. "They are all important, but if I have to pick the least important I would say the bedtime issue." "What are the kids' bedtimes, and what do you know about their bedtimes at John's house?" She answered that she enforced a 9:30 bedtime and seldom made exceptions. She said that Becky had told her that on weekends John let them stay up as long as they wanted and that on weekdays he let them go to bed as late as 10:30. "That's not true!" John protested.

"On weekdays I try to get them to bed by 9:30. Every now and then I let them stay up for something special, but it's only once in a while. And I'm not even willing to discuss weekends. They can sleep late in the morning and there is nothing wrong with it."

They argued for a short time, and then I asked if there was any rule John might agree to with respect to bedtime. He replied that he would be willing to try to adhere to a 9:30 bedtime during the week but not on weekends. I asked Maria if she could live with that, and she said yes even though she would have reservations.

COMMENTARY: Bedtime is one of numerous subjective practices that parents develop over time, based on their own personal biases and experience, and often on their schedules. These are relatively easy to resolve by encouraging each party to compromise a little. If one party does not feel particularly strongly, it is wise to accommodate and respect the party who does feel strongly. Other issues are not as easy.

I asked John about giving Ritalin to Jeb.

"I have never said that I won't give him the medicine, but the doctor never said to use it when Jeb is not in school. In general, I don't think it's a good thing to give these medications unless it's absolutely necessary."

"Have you asked the doctor?" I inquired.

"No, I haven't. Maria always takes Jeb to the doctor, and I've never met him."

I asked him whether he would meet with the doctor and abide by the doctor's judgment, and he agreed that he would. I asked Maria if that was acceptable to her, and so we moved on.

COMMENTARY: Most parents agree about medical treatment for their children. They choose a physician, take the child when he or she is sick or needs a checkup, and do what the doctor tells them to do. But occasionally we see people who are deeply invested in a particular viewpoint. One of my clients, a chiropractor, was strongly opposed to vaccinating children. His wife had gone along reluctantly while they were married, but now she wanted the children to be vaccinated. This caused intense conflict because both genuinely believed that they were fighting for the health of the children. I strongly encourage people to identify a pediatrician acceptable to both and to abide by the doctor's advice. If a doctor prescribes medicine, each parent is obliged to carry through. I have seen too many court battles caused by one parent's deviating from medical advice because that parent had decided that his or her expertise exceeded that of the doctor. I strongly discourage such behavior. I find that even when one or both of the parents are devotees of "alternative medicine," they can usually find a physician whose approaches are compatible with both their viewpoints.

We then took up the motorcycle and the snowmobile issues. I asked them if they could agree that the children would always wear generally acceptable protective gear when riding bikes, horses, rollerblades, skateboards, or any vehicle in which they were exposed to injury. John said that he would. "Well, why didn't they have helmets on when they were on the snowmobile?" asked Maria. John answered:

"That was a one-time exception that won't happen again. We had an opportunity to try three snowmobiles one day, and we didn't have helmets with us. I felt the conditions were not too dangerous, so I made an exception for the few minutes that the ride lasted. I have no intention of letting it happen again."

Maria then raised the question of the motorcycle, and John became angry.

"You have never liked motorcycles, but they are an important part of what I like to do, and you're not going to stop me from sharing that with the kids. There is nothing wrong with riding motorcycles if you are careful, and I have never had an accident, because I am careful."

But Maria was adamant.

"Motorcycles are 20 times more likely to get you killed than cars. It doesn't matter how careful you are. If some crazy driver comes along, you're dead. If you want to kill yourself, that's up to you, but you are not taking the kids with you!"

COMMENTARY: My experience suggests several observations about gender differences and parenting. Of course there are exceptions, but I have found that men are generally more risk-tolerant than women and tend to be more insistent that their children be allowed to take greater risks. Risk taking, autonomy, independence, and mastery are often more important to men's identity than they are to the identity of women. And if the child is a boy, many men worry lest the child turn out to be a sissy. So, it is not uncommon that fathers and mothers disagree about what is and is not safe. Although there are some women who are physically bolder than their husbands, the issue of physical safety for the children is more likely to be asserted by mothers than by fathers. So, when Maria and John square off about permission to ride on John's motorcycle, that is the script being played out. Again, I urge clients to consider the transaction cost. What is it worth to him? And what does it cost her?

I asked John how central motorcycle riding was to him. "It's not the most important thing in the world, but I find it thrilling, and I want to share it with Jeb." I asked him whether he understood how frightened it made Maria. "She's always been frightened about the bike, and I've never been able to get her to come with me." So, I asked him if, given that history, he believed that Maria's resistance to Jeb's motorcycle riding was caused by real distress or whether she was just trying to thwart him. "No, she has always been scared of the bike, and this is nothing new." I asked him if he could conceive of keeping Jeb off the motorcycle not because Maria was right but because she was so frightened that it wasn't worth causing her this degree of grief over what was simply an enjoyable pastime.

"But what about the principle of the thing? Does this mean that every time she doesn't like what I'm doing she can tell me what to do?"

I turned to Maria and asked her if this meant that she was trying to tell John what to do. She replied:

"No, John. I am really terrified about this. If you could accommodate me, I would really be grateful."

In the end, John agreed that Jeb would not be invited to ride on the motorcycle until he was 15 years old. And John's agreement was reframed as an accommodation to Maria's fears rather than a submission to her will.

COMMENTARY: Just because one is getting divorced does not mean that one can give up one's humanity with respect to the other spouse. When there is an agreement on something related to risk tolerance, the degree of distress caused to one is a legitimate factor for the other to consider without worrying whether this is submission to domination and control. That does not mean that one should always agree to do it the other's way but that the other's feelings are still an appropriate basis of cost–benefit analysis. The payoff is that it works both ways and that one can expect the other to reciprocate when strong feelings are at stake. This is not a matter of rights. It is a matter of retaining a working relationship in which both parents feel respected.

THE THERAPIST'S ROLE IN CUSTODY AND PARENTING DECISIONS

Most of the conflict that occurs over children is not related to custody struggles. Rather, it is related to disagreements about how to manage the children in two households. Disagreements over homework, discipline, bedtimes, nutrition, household chores, risk tolerance, spending, and pickup and delivery of the children are the commonplace conflicts that, left unattended, can sour the parenting relationship. Therapists can and should play a major role in helping parents manage these conflicts. Generally, parents need someone to normalize the situation and to calm things down. Anxious parents and guilty parents can easily blow these issues out of proportion. More often than not, the transaction costs of these issues far outweigh the issue that parents believe to be at stake. If a child is put to bed later than the other parent wants, if the child eats hotdogs and cheeseburgers at the other household, if the child does not quite get his or her homework done some nights, or if a child is allowed to watch a movie that the other parent disapproves of are all issues that I have seen cause appearances in court. And not one of these issues was worth the cost in dollars, or the resultant alienation between the parents, or the wear and tear on the children. There are so many messages to people encouraging them to fight in the "best interests of the child" that the forest is rapidly lost in the trees. What we need is a professional who counsels calm and peace and who teaches that children can adapt to different routines and regimes in two households.

It is useful for therapists working with divorcing couples to familiarize themselves with practical tips that will make the arrangement smoother. For example, kids are notorious for forgetting items as they move from household to household–clothing, toys, sports equipment, or homework supplies. So, it helps to have a full complement in each household, if possible. Some schools are accustomed to dealing with children of divorced parents and are willing to provide two sets of textbooks, one for each household.

Therapists can also underscore the importance of honoring the separation agreement as it applies to children. If a father is to pick up a child at 6 P.M. he needs to be there at 6 P.M. If there is an occasional tardy arrival, he needs to call, explain, and apologize. Parents need to protect the integrity of the relationship between the child and the other parent. Primary residential mothers need to ensure that father's time with the children is not undermined by plans made at the last minute that interfere with the child's time with the father. The real issue here is one of simple humanity. In the struggle that is divorce, it is very easy for a spouse to forget that the other deserves to be treated with respect and humanity. Perhaps therapists have become a last resort as teachers of humanity.

The other critical task for therapists is to help people manage the transition when one or both former spouses become involved in relationships with new significant others. This is most problematic the first time the other spouse becomes involved, as this may trigger intense feelings of jealousy, even in the partner who initiated the divorce. But, because people are reluctant to admit that they are jealous, it is common for that emotion to be masked as some issue involving the child. This is a potentially damaging situation, and it needs to be firmly addressed by the therapist. Again, it is a matter of normalizing and calming down. The emotion of jealousy is normal, but it should not be allowed to interfere with the adaptation of the entire family to divorce. This adaptation typically involves the building of new intimate relationships. Of course, the therapist must also help parents address the potential anger, insecurity, and fear that children often experience when their parents begin dating, and especially when parents have started a new relationship. So, in all these situations–some that arise early in the divorce and some that arise after the divorce is over–a proactive role by the therapist can significantly enhance the successful completion of the tasks of divorce and can enable the family to achieve the goal of a good divorce.

Summary of the Therapist's Role in Facilitating Parenting Arrangements

- Facilitate decision making by helping the client distinguish between "major" and "minor" parenting decisions.
- Provide practical tips to facilitate the parenting structure.
- Encourage flexibility and creativity.
- Reinforce the client's commitment to the agreed-upon parenting schedule.
- Proactively address emotions that arise from new relationships.
- Address emotions and resentment toward the former spouse.
- Remind the client to engage in behaviors that facilitate cooperation, even in the face of unresolved anger or resentment.
- Remind the client that cooperation between the parents promotes good adjustment to the divorce among the children.

10 Child Support and Alimony

Two of the most contentious issues of divorce are child support and alimony. Property division is the most difficult issue for a few wealthy couples. But most middle-class couples do not have enough property to argue over division. For these couples, child support and alimony are the most difficult issues to negotiate. And alimony is one that gives men the hardest time. In this chapter, I want to help the therapist understand the issues and provide useful ways to counsel clients about support. We will begin by talking about child support and then discuss alimony.

CHILD SUPPORT DEFINED

Child support is paid by one spouse to the other as a contribution to pay the children's expenses. Supporting children is the responsibility of both parents until the children are legally emancipated. All states have support guidelines that allocate responsibility between the mother and father in proportion to their incomes. There is considerable variation from state to state, and in my opinion none of the state guidelines for child support that I have seen is adequate. Child support is usually paid to the parent of primary residence by the other parent. So, if the children are living principally with the mother, the father is expected to pay her child support. And if the children live primarily with the father, the mother would be expected to pay child support to him. Although that happens on occasion, by far the most common arrangement is that the father pays child support. Child support is not taxable income. It is paid with after-tax dollars. One earns the money, pays taxes, and then pays child support from what remains.

Child support is paid until "emancipation," which is defined variously in different states. All states consider a child emancipated at age

18 or graduation from high school, but some states defer emancipation if the child goes to college. So, in New Jersey, for example, children who go to college directly from high school are eligible for child support and can expect help from parents with college expenses. The New Jersey courts have held that it is unrealistic to consider a child emancipated at 18. North Carolina, on the other hand, regards children emancipated at 18 and makes no demand on parents to assist with college.

HOW MUCH CHILD SUPPORT SHOULD BE PAID?

There are two ways to think about how much child support should be paid. The first is to follow the child support guidelines of the state of residence. Fifteen years ago, the federal government required all states to establish minimum guidelines for their courts to follow when awarding child support. The legislation was caused by judges who ordered ridiculously low child support and left the primary parent struggling to support the children. The legislation did not establish the same guidelines for all states but required each state to construct its own guidelines. States courts appointed committees to recommend guidelines to the court. In most states, the guidelines apply up to some maximum level of family income, and then discretion reverts to the court beyond that level. The guidelines are *minimum* levels of support, based on the relative incomes of the parents. Judges will not permit lower support unless the couple provides justification.

There are several problems with child support guidelines. First is that the standard of living established by the guidelines is politically influenced. It is shaped by the values of the lawyers who serve on the committees. Few lawyers are sophisticated in economics or in statistics. And many are responsive to various constituencies such as women's groups and fathers' rights groups that campaign for higher or lower standards. The result is considerable variation in the amount of child support paid from state to state. And the amount of support your state guidelines require your clients to pay may be woefully inadequate to meet their children's needs. Even though guidelines are supposed to establish minimum standards, few lawyers and judges inquire whether the application of the guidelines in a particular case provides enough support. Many lawyers are disinclined to think beyond the guidelines—so, for them, the minimum guidelines also become the maximum guidelines.

A second problem is that the way the guidelines have evolved in many states actually promotes conflict between parents. When they were first applied, the formulas were simple. The needs of the children were calculated, and child support was determined as a fixed percentage of the payer's income or was determined by applying a straight ratio of the husband's income to the wife's income. So, if he earned $1,000 a week and she earned $500 a week, he would pay two-thirds of the amount needed by the children. Although there were some conceptual inconsistencies in these formulas, they were simple and could be calculated in seconds.

But, as time went on, the committees in charge of formulating the guidelines got more sophisticated. In particular, they responded to the lobbying of fathers' rights groups, which wanted support standards reduced in general and more specifically sought reduced support when children spent more time with their fathers. Conceptually, the argument had merit in that children spending more time with their fathers generally lowered costs to the mothers and raised them for the fathers, thus requiring some adjustment. But this caused several problems. Calculating adjustments sometimes required formulas so complex that computer programs were needed. After all, how do you really calculate the impact on household expenses when a child spends one more night a week at the father's house and one less at the mother's house? How do you calculate the change in utilities or food bills? Many expenses are fixed and do not vary, while others vary with time spent. So, the result was guidelines that are extremely complex, require more lawyer time, and produce higher legal fees but not much else.

But the biggest problem with complicated guidelines is that they connect the amount of support paid to the amount of time the child spends with the father. So, if the mother is the parent of primary residence, she gets less support if the child spends 2 nights a week with the father than if the child spends 1 night a week with the father. As a consequence, we often find in negotiations that the mother is suspicious that the only reason the father wants more time with the kids is because he wants to reduce financial support. On the other hand, the father believes that the mother withholds the children because she wants more support. Linking the amount of time the child spends with the father to the amount of support paid has produced a minor disaster in the courts. It promotes cynicism and leads lawyers to suggest to their clients that the other parent is motivated only by money rather than the needs of the child. Some lawyers counsel clients to seek more or less time with the children simply to minimize or maximize child support. This change has served lawyers well but divorcing families very poorly. It has made it more difficult to resolve divorces, has prolonged litigation unduly, and has enriched lawyers.

Finally, the guidelines may have little to do with the way your clients have raised their children. Suppose they spend $1,000 a month on their children and the support guidelines, based on their family income, only provide $700 per month. Following the child support the guidelines will result in insufficient support. Child support guidelines were intended as minimums for people who cannot agree and assume an adversarial relationship between the spouses. They assume and promote a bad divorce.

ALTERNATIVES TO CHILD SUPPORT GUIDELINES: BUDGET-BASED CHILD SUPPORT

An alternative to child support guidelines is to prepare accurate budgets for both households that identify the expenses attributable to the children and then together to reconcile how the income is allocated to each family member. This requires more work but avoids the arbitrariness of the guidelines.

Case Study: Barry and Barbara

Barry and Barbara have two children, ages 10 and 7. Barry is a marketing executive and earns $110,000 a year. Barbara is a paralegal and earns $55,000 a year. The couple is divorcing. They have decided that the children will live primarily with Barbara, because Barry's work requires him to travel frequently. They have agreed that their budgets are as follows:

	Barbara	Barry
Children's expenses	$2,700	$400
Individual costs	$3,000	$3,000
Total monthly expenses	$5,700	$3,400
Take-home pay	$3,575	$6,700
Monthly deficit/surplus	$2,125	$3,300

Let's look at the different ways that Barry and Barbara can calculate child support. Barbara does not seek alimony, so that is not an issue.

Child Support Guidelines

Barry and Barbara consult the guidelines and find that for two children in families with total income of $165,000 a year, guidelines project the total cost of children to be $2,200 monthly. The guidelines allocate the cost proportionate to income, and as Barry earns two-thirds of the total family income, his projected child support would be two-thirds of $2,200, or $1,467 per month. His lawyer has told him that he does not have to pay more than that if he does not want to. So, if Barry pays the guidelines support of $1,467, Barbara's monthly deficit of $2,125 will only be reduced to $658. Note that Barbara and Barry have each calculated their individual costs at $3,000 per month.

Where is Barbara to make up her deficit? She will either have to reduce her own standard of living or reduce the children's standard of living, or both. And where will this leave Barry? He has a budget surplus of $3,300 from which he pays $1,467, leaving what is now a monthly surplus of $1,833. His budget is fully funded, while the budgets for Barbara and the children are reduced approximately 12%.

Real Costs of the Children, with Pro-Rata Allocation

The first alternative is to calculate support based on the actual cost of the children and apply the ratio of income earned by each party. The total cost of the children has been calculated at $3,100, of which $2,700 is incurred in Barbara's house and $400 is incurred in Barry's house. If Barry were to pay two-thirds of this, he would pay a total of $2,067, of which he is already paying $400 in his own house. So, he would pay Barbara the difference, $1,667. Now Barbara has a deficit of $458 a month while Barry has a surplus of $1,633. Barbara still has a difficult choice. If she is to spend the $3,000 on herself that she and Barry each calculated as their own personal expenses, then she must manage her $458 per month deficit by unilaterally reducing the children's standard of living. Or, if she is unwilling to cut the children's consumption, she will have to cut her own consumption by $458 each month and, in effect, give that to the children. In either case, she will be resentful watching Barry enjoy a surplus while she absorbs what she regards as a disproportionate share of the children's expenses.

The real problem is that allocating child support based on proportion of earnings is unfair. Thus, if a wife earns one-quarter of the income, she should pay one-quarter of the support. But why is this fair? The assumption is that people should pay relative to their ability to pay and that by allocating support based on percentage of family income earned we are allocating based on ability to pay. But when we look at how this applies to Barry and Barbara, we are left with some troubling inconsistencies. If Barbara and Barry each need $3,000 monthly for themselves, what really is their capacity to contribute to the children? Barbara brings home only $3,575 a month and needs $3,000 for herself. If we tell her to pay one-third of the children's costs, which is $1,033, it does not relate to her ability to pay. This system leaves Barbara with a deficit, while it leaves Barry with a surplus.

To be fair, we would measure ability to contribute to the children by what is left over after each has paid his or her own essential costs–in other words, their discretionary income. After paying $3,000 for herself, Barbara has $575 left each month. After paying $3,000 for himself, Barry has $3,700 left each month. What happens if we base our allocation on the percentage of discretionary income?

Barry's discretionary income per month	$3,700
Barbara's discretionary income per month	$575
Total discretionary income	$4,275
Barry's percentage of discretionary income	86.5%
Barbara's percentage of discretionary income	13.5%

Now, let's apply this to the couple's budgets and see what we get. The total cost of the children is $3,100, of which Barry should pay 86.5%, or $2,681. He is already paying $400 in his own house, so his payment to Barbara should be $2,261.

	Barbara	Barry
Expenses	$5,700	$3,400
Income	$3,575	$6,700
Child support	$2,261	$2,261
Surplus	$136	$1,039

With this allocation, the children's budgets are fully funded in each household. Barbara's needs are fully funded. She has a small budget surplus of $136, while Barry has a larger budget surplus of $1,039. Barry is still wealthier than Barbara, a reflection of his greater income. They have not been made equal. But child support has been allocated fairly between them. This method of equitable child support allocation is not reflected in any of the child support guidelines of which I am aware. I know of few lawyers who use this approach. But it is the only way to obtain a fair result. Lawyers don't encourage this method, nor do judges in court. So, people do not do it. Nevertheless I believe that a good divorce requires such an analysis.

Whether or not you as a therapist are willing to be involved in matters as concrete as child support calculations will vary, depending on your own strengths and preferences. But it is important that you understand the different approaches so that you can understand what is going on and the impact this has on your client's feelings and sense of fairness.

HEALTH AND LIFE INSURANCE

Child support agreements usually specify which parent will provide health insurance for the children. Typically, at least one partner who is employed can cover the children through his or her employer's group health insurance at a reasonable cost. This makes sense when it is possible, because it saves money and usually provides better coverage than do individual plans. The extra cost of the children's premium is a negotiable item. The agreement should also specify how the spouses will pay for uninsured medical and dental expenses. For the most part, these are limited to copayments for medical treatment, but they may also involve considerable expense for dental work and orthodontics, or for counseling. These expenses should be apportioned between the two spouses in a manner similar to how they allocate child support.

The spouses should also agree on life insurance to protect the children if one of the parents dies. People should estimate the total projected support to be paid until the child is emancipated and provide an amount of term life insurance to cover that. Ideally, both parents provide life insurance for the children, with the surviving parent designated as trustee. If the father dies, the children will be solely reliant on their mother, and she should not have to go, hat in hand, seeking money from former in-laws every time she needs to spend on the children. Unless she is obviously incompetent in the management of money, she should be the trustee. Term insurance is usually the only sensible way to get life insurance when cash flow is tight. Universal and whole-life policies are really savings programs, and few divorcing couples can afford to save money in this way.

COLLEGE

Couples are frequently worried about paying for college for the children. This is urgent if the children are nearing college age, but less urgent if the children are younger. The obligation to contribute to college expenses varies from state to state. But if the parents want the children to attend college, how should they negotiate this? They are reluctant to leave the matter undetermined, but they also do not want to bind themselves to pay unlimited amounts for college. The majority of children attend college at state-supported institutions that cost only a third as much as prestigious private institutions. But an open-ended commitment to pay for any college can leave parents financially ruined as the enter their later years. Because these expenses are paid with after-tax dollars, few parents can afford to give their children carte blanche to choose any school they want.

There are a few important principles to apply here. First, if parents choose to commit to paying for college in their separation agreement, they should limit the obligation to the cost of room, board, and tuition at a state school for a state resident. If the child chooses a more expensive college, he or she can take out student loans, work, or negotiate other arrangements with the parents. Divorce stretches the cash flow of most people. Being able to save money while paying alimony or child support is unlikely. If the parents have a lot of assets, they can put some aside for college before dividing the assets between them. For those who have the money, this is ideal. But those without the money will have to manage college expenses as the need arises and agree that each of them will contribute relative to his or her ability to pay. This should be discussed as the child enters the junior year of high school.

Some Principles for Thinking about Child Support

- Supporting children is the responsibility of both parents relative to their ability to pay.
- Child support should be based on rigorous budgeting for the households of both parents.
- State-mandated child support guidelines may be inadequate to the needs of the children.
- Gross disparities in the living standards of the two households will likely breed resentment and lack of cooperation over the long run.

THE PSYCHOLOGY OF SUPPORT

Paying child support often troubles the men who are paying. Many feel that they are paying money to their ex-wives rather than to their children. Some want to spend the money directly, paying for clothing and other items, rather than through child support paid to the mother. But if the child is living principally with the mother and the mother administers the financial affairs of the children, having the father pay bills directly introduces too much complexity that inevitably causes trouble. Simplicity is elegant. Men need to be helped to manage the feelings that they have lost control because they are not provided with monthly accountings. There is no practical remedy for such feelings, and the court will not require the mother to make accountings to the father.

A problem often observed in support discussions is the tendency of the mother to assume the role of economic bargaining agent for the children. This is most likely in traditional arrangements, in which the children live with the mother, the father pays support, and the mother spends the money on the children. When discussing support, there is usually vigorous discussion about how much money is really necessary. We usually find the mother arguing in favor of additional spending on the child and the father arguing for less. The mother tends to slide into the role of the children's agent, and the husband slides into the role of resentful provider. This is a bad psychological position for both, because it positions her as the good parent and the husband as the bad guy.

To avoid this trap, the spouses must be encouraged to follow a disciplined budgeting process. If the two have jointly calculated what the children cost, then any reductions in the children's budgets must be decided by both parents. If there is a deficit, any extra money to be spent on the children has to be offset by specific reductions in the budgets of the parents. By continually referring to the budgets, they achieve financial discipline for the entire family and avoid the trap that arises when the wife poses as the only parent dedicated to the children.

It is natural that parents want to avoid depriving their children of the amenities of life. Often we find one or both parents arguing that the adults should do without whenever it is a question of reducing the standard of living of the children. It is easy for the welfare of the children to become a pious invocation intended to embarrass the other parent into further concessions on behalf of the children. So, some people who cannot afford private school for their children keep them in private school even though it wrecks the family finances, because they feel too guilty to impose change on the children. Parents do their children no favors by casting the entire family into financial chaos. As I have noted so many times throughout this book, divorce is about change. All members of the family have to absorb their share of change and dislocation. All may have to accept spending reductions for a while. It is shortsighted when parents sacrifice their own basic needs to preserve amenities for the children. Children thrive only to the extent that their parents thrive. Assume that all needs could be ranked on a scale of 1 to 10. Having enough food to eat is a 10, but eating lobster is a 1. Having proper clothing is a 10, but having a particular pair of designer jeans is a 1. In principle, no one in the family should get level 4 needs met until everyone else in the family has had level 5 needs met. The family needs to share in good fortune and less fortune more or less equally.

RICH HOUSE, POOR HOUSE

When couples have joint custody and the children live half of the time with each parent, child support discussions require careful consideration. The parents each have to maintain a fully equipped home for the children. Each child needs a separate bedroom, and each home needs a full complement of computers, toys, books, games, and other equipment that modern children desire. So, the total cost for two completely equipped homes exceeds the total cost when one home is primary and the other is used by the children just on weekends. Real joint custody is more expensive than joint legal custody.

Joint custody tends to fare very poorly when there is a great disparity in the living standards of the two homes. Children quickly figure out where the goodies are, and their behavior may soon reflect their preference. Managing the hard feelings of the parent in the "poor" home then becomes difficult. What this means is that joint custody costs more, and the child support guidelines are a very poor guide for making joint custody work. Let us now turn to alimony, often the most difficult subject of divorce.

WHAT IS ALIMONY?

Alimony is support paid by one spouse to another. Occasionally, wives pay alimony to husbands, but these are exceptional situations. Generally, when alimony is paid, it is husbands paying alimony to wives. Alimony differs from child support in several ways. First, it is paid with pretax dollars. The payer gets to deduct alimony from gross income before calculating his taxes. The recipient treats the alimony as taxable income. This may have some significant financial implications, as we shall see later. We are concerned with three issues in alimony discussions: whether alimony should be paid at all, how much alimony should be paid, and for how long it should be paid.

SHOULD THERE BE ALIMONY?

Several important factors influence whether alimony should be paid in a particular divorce. Most important are need and capacity. Alimony is not an issue if the two spouses have approximately the same income. So, if a husband earns $75,000 a year and his wife earns $67,000 a year, it is not an alimony case. Alimony requires a significant disparity in incomes. There is no clear threshold of disparity that distinguishes the alimony case from the nonalimony case, but as a rule of thumb unless one spouse's income is at least 50% greater than the other's, there is probably no alimony due. When there is a significant disparity in incomes, alimony serves to reduce it. But there is no premise that the two incomes must be equalized. There are a few conditions in which we consider trying to equalize household incomes, but we will come to those later.

TYPES OF ALIMONY

There are generally three types of alimony, each defined by how long alimony is to be paid and under what conditions it terminates. The first type is called rehabilitative alimony, which is intended to support a spouse until she (or he) is able to support herself. Rehabilitative alimony assumes that the recipient is obligated to work for her own support and assumes that, once she is employed at some defined level of income, alimony will end. The duration of rehabilitative alimony is determined by how long it will take the wife to complete training or other credentialing activity so that she can qualify for employment. The range of possibilities here is broad. A high school graduate who has been married for 6 years might have rehabilitative alimony to qualify her for a year of training to become a secretary or a paralegal. Or a wife with a college degree might qualify for support through graduate school to get a law degree or an MSW or other degree. The couple must agree on what is a reasonable goal under the circumstances. Rehabilitative alimony can also be paid to supplement the salary of a woman who has been out of the workforce for some years and needs time to reestablish herself in a career for which she has the credentials but needs to restore her seniority in the industry.

When discussing rehabilitative alimony, we need to specify the goals and objectives of rehabilitation. We must decide in advance the income level to which the wife is to be restored or the credential she will achieve before she is regarded as economically rehabilitated and ready for economic independence.

The second type of alimony, and the most traditional, is "permanent" alimony–sometimes mistakenly called "lifetime" alimony. This alimony is paid until the wife remarries or one of the spouses dies. I put permanent in quotation marks because nothing is really permanent. Better to call it "alimony of indeterminate duration"–but the law has called it permanent. This type of alimony recalls the days when women were expected to be traditional homemakers and not expected to assume equal roles in the workplace. Such alimony is paid until another husband comes along to support the wife. Long ago, when there was only fault-based divorce, such alimony was paid only when it was proved that the misconduct of the husband was the cause of the divorce. If the wife was at fault, she received no alimony. Although permanent alimony was originally a commonplace feature of fault-based divorce, it has persisted into no-fault divorce.

The third type of alimony is alimony for a term of years, either negotiated by the parties or imposed by the court. Alimony for a period of years is generally used as a compromise between permanent alimony and rehabilitative alimony. Whereas a long-term marriage would be expected to require permanent alimony and a short-term marriage would support only rehabilitative alimony, alimony for a period of years is designed to accommodate marriages of medium duration in which the courts are reluctant to impose an indeterminate alimony but are equally hesitant to limit alimony to rehabilitative support. Whereas there is an inherent logic to both permanent and rehabilitative alimony, there is no such logic that attaches to alimony for a period of years. We have no assurance that the wife will be able to support herself at the end of this period. If alimony is negotiated for 10 years, for example, it simply means that the wife will assume the risk that she will not be remarried or that she will not be able to support herself at the standard of living that she seeks. Alimony for a fixed period is more about how risk is distributed than it is about anything else. Not all states have this type of alimony. All states will enforce a settlement agreement that specifies alimony for a period of years, but not all states authorize courts to impose such limits on alimony.

CHANGES IN CIRCUMSTANCES

After a divorce is over, changes in the lives of the former partners and their children may sometimes require the renegotiation of the support agreement. The division of assets is not subject to change or renegotiation. Once property is divided, the division is final. But the issues related to custody, child support, and alimony are subject to change if the circumstances of the parties change dramatically. This body of law is complicated, and there are dramatic differences from state to state.

A persistent issue arises when the income of either party changes dramatically. When one spouse receives alimony and child support, the other may be concerned about having to pay the same amount of support even if his (or her) income decreases precipitously. He seeks assurance that the support will be reduced if such a decrease in income occurs. He also wants to know how a dramatic increase in the income of the wife might affect his support obligations. Alimony ceases if she remarries. But what happens if she is single and inherits a large sum of money or if her career takes off and her pay increases dramatically? The spouse receiving support also worries. Will her (or his) income be secure if the ex quits his (or her) job? And if he gets a big promotion, will she receive an increase in alimony and child support? These questions about changes in circumstances probably generate more post-divorce conflict than any other issue.

Although the law varies from state to state, there are some principles that generally apply. First, men paying support will usually be granted relief by the court when, through no fault of their own, they suffer a long-term and significant reduction in income. This was the case for many people employed in the securities industry who lost their jobs when the stock market plateaued in the late 1990s and contracted at the turn of the 21st century. Many were unemployed for years and were grateful to find any employment, even if it paid much less than they had previously earned. The courts will usually reduce the support obligations of such men, because it would be cruel and unrealistic to require them to pay the same level of support established when they had much higher income. Similarly, a big increase in the wife's income by promotion or inheritance may require adjustments such as an increase in the wife's contribution to supporting the children or even a reduction in alimony. Lawyers are forever trying to write clauses into contracts that make the agreement hard or impossible to change. Some attempts are successful; the courts overturn others. As a therapist, you cannot possibly stay abreast of such developments. Just be aware that some couples may get into contention because they are trying to immunize the agreement against change. Sometimes the amount of energy devoted to this issue defies common sense when the changes one partner seeks to avoid are remote. In divorce, the therapist who counsels common sense will never lead a client astray.

THE EMOTIONAL IMPLICATIONS OF ALIMONY

People going through divorce are often distressed by the negotiation of alimony. When alimony is not an issue, the divorce is usually fairly simple. But, for example, when husbands are asked to continue to support a woman with whom he no longer has a life, he is likely to be resistant and resentful. (While I recognize that, on occasion, women end up paying alimony to their former husbands after divorce, in the vast majority of cases in which alimony comes up, it is the husband who pays it.)

When the wife is the initiator and the husband doesn't want the divorce, he may be infuriated by her demand for alimony. As one of my clients told me, "She is leaving me and will no longer provide any services such as caring for the house, cooking and cleaning, arranging our social life, and taking care of me, not to mention sex. So, why do I have to continue to support her?"

To some extent, alimony seems unfair and hardly consistent with gender equality. In large measure alimony is still a creature of historical circumstance, and many of its principles are inconsistent with contemporary norms. For example, alimony automatically ends when a woman remarries. So, a woman is rewarded with alimony for devoting her most vigorous years to raising a family and maintaining a household for her successful husband. She "earned" the support, and it would be unfair to cast her out, or on her own resources. Then, why end it if she remarries? What if she marries a man whose income is low and who cannot support her? What if he is paying alimony and child support to his ex-wife and barely has enough left to care for himself? Why, when the wife is "passed" off to another man, is the first husband relieved of responsibility whether the new husband can support her or not? This historical rule is not economically relevant to the present. Nevertheless, lawyers universally express horror when I suggest that alimony ought not to end automatically upon remarriage. Men fear that the alimony would be used to support another man or, horror of horrors, "I am supposed to support her while some other guy is sleeping with her? Are you nuts?"

The legal norms for alimony may often feel unfair and outdated. So, what should your clients do? I encourage the use of alimony to achieve justice between spouses. The amount and duration of alimony should be sufficient that both partners can lead successful new lives. We maintain a vision of successful divorce that uses family resources to maximize success for all members of the family rather than using money as a vehicle of retribution or the vindication of agendas resulting from the failed marriage.

Most states have modernized alimony to the extent that most judges are not interested in linking alimony to marital fault or misconduct. From a therapeutic perspective, such a link is unproductive for families. But there are some states in which marital misconduct, particularly infidelity, can be used as a basis for awarding or denying alimony. In North Carolina, where I practice, as well as in several other Deep South states, adultery is an absolute bar to alimony. Even when the affair occurs after many years of emotional neglect, it can still be used to punish the wife. I regard this as unfortunate and will usually decline cases in which the husband seeks to do this. Just because the law allows it does not mean people have to do it that way. A decent divorce does not include vindictive behavior.

Case Study: Phil and Janie

Phil and Janie are negotiating their separation agreement. Phil is a physician, and Janie has been a homemaker for 20 years, after an early career as a nurse. She never particularly liked being a nurse, and when Phil started to succeed in his practice, she was happy to give up nursing and devote herself to making a home for Phil and their three children. Phil is now 59, and Janie is 51. Their marriage had eroded for many years, and 6 months ago Janie told Phil that she wanted a divorce. She had pleaded with him for years to devote more time to her and the family but felt that he always put his practice first. Phil resented her critique because he believed that as an infectious disease specialist he had no choice but to work the hours necessary to serve his patients. All successful physicians put in long hours, and Phil believed that Janie was unfair in her demands. The couple had never been able to resolve this issue, and Janie had gradually built a life for herself that had less and less to do with Phil. She had made her own friends, become active in volunteer projects in the community and at their church, and devoted herself to supervising the three children, the youngest of whom was now in college.

When Janie told Phil that she wanted a divorce, he was shocked at first. But as he thought about it he became angry with Janie. He had always worked as hard as he could to provide for his family. Now, when he was just approaching the time that he might slow down a little and be able to relax more often, here was Janie bailing out. It felt as if she had used him to get the kids raised, and now that they were off on their own she was done with him. Now she was going to go play and expect him to continue to work and support her. He felt used and abandoned by her.

Although they had decided to try mediation, he had only agreed because he had heard how lawyers loved to litigate when doctors were involved and he feared that legal costs would get out of hand if they did a litigated divorce. He was hoping to avoid an ugly fight but was nevertheless angry and indignant about the divorce.

Janie had consulted with several lawyers. All the lawyers had told her that, because she was an economically dependent spouse, she was entitled to receive alimony from Phil even though she was the one who wanted a divorce. Phil earned about $300,000 a year and had the capacity to support her. They had been married for 27 years, and long-term marriages such as hers, she was told, justified permanent alimony–meaning that Phil would have to support her until she remarried, one of them died, or the court allowed him to retire. Not only was she entitled to receive alimony, but also under the laws of New Jersey where this case occurred she was entitled to receive enough alimony to allow her to live "in the manner to which she was accustomed" so long as Phil earned enough income to afford that level of support.

Phil had also consulted lawyers and had been told that, indeed, he could expect to pay alimony and that considering his income, the length of the marriage, and the fact that Janie did not have a career, he could end up paying as much as one-third of his income to her.

> "You mean to tell me that I have to work 60 hours a week and she gets a third of my income for doing nothing? How is that fair? She no longer has to do anything for me. I lose the benefit of her services as a homemaker and companion, but she gets to receive a big chunk of my income as long as she wants. That's outrageous!"

His lawyer had advised him that he could fight it in court but that it was very unlikely that a judge would deny her alimony. They could struggle in court to keep the alimony to a minimum, but the law in these cases suggested that she would get substantial alimony.

> "Well, doesn't she have any obligation to work? She is a trained nurse. I'm sure she would need some retraining, but at most she would need a year of training and could easily earn $40,000 a year or more in any hospital around here. Why is she able to retire and sit on her butt while I'm out busting mine?"

Again the lawyer could only provide infuriatingly vague answers.

"Well, it would depend on what judge we got. Some judges might decide that she had been a homemaker for so long that she didn't have to resume a career at 51, particularly one for which her skills were no longer current. We might get a judge who expected her to earn something, and we might even convince the judge to impute some income to her. That means that the judge would assume that she was able to earn money and would reduce the alimony to reflect that. But remember that the standard of living we're talking about is based on what you earn, and even though the judge required her to work, the $30,000 or $40,000 she could earn would only reduce your obligation. She would never be expected to live on that salary. I hate to tell you, but you are swimming upstream on this one."

Phil did not like what he was hearing.

"But what about retirement? We had always talked about my retiring at 60, getting a smaller house on the water, and enjoying life before I got too old. What happens if I retire next year as I had planned?"

Again, the lawyer's answer was not comforting.

"You can retire, but that does not mean that you would be excused from paying alimony. If she is able to earn enough income from her share of the assets to support herself, you might find a judge who would let you out. But remember that you are going to be talking to a judge who earns less than half of what you do and who can't retire until 65. In this state, a voluntary reduction of alimony does not usually support an application to reduce alimony. We do have some cases that suggest that if you retire at 65 the court *will regard that as reasonable and reduce alimony. But there are no guarantees, even then.*"

An incredulous Phil recapitulated:

> "So, let me get this straight. I can't retire when we planned, but she can retire now. I have to work as hard as ever, but she doesn't have to do anything. She doesn't have to work, but I do. She doesn't have to do anything for me, but I have to support her. Tell me, where is the justice in this?"

The lawyer could only shrug his shoulders.

Alimony and Anger

Phil's sentiments are not unusual and reveal almost all the issues that arise in a negotiation about alimony.

1. *"She is leaving me, so why do I have to support her? I didn't do anything wrong. Why do I get punished because she decides to end the marriage?"* It is understandable that some men experience the requirement to pay alimony as punishment. But punishment no longer has a place in the modern divorce. With the shift to no-fault divorce, alimony is no longer linked to misconduct, so it must be based on general concepts of equity and fairness. Marriage is a joint venture in which each spouse contributes and shares in the good and bad fortunes of the marriage. Although husbands are more often the primary breadwinners, or at least tend to outearn their wives, the domestic contribution of the wife is regarded as her contribution to the family. The awarding of alimony is increasingly influenced by general principles of contract. Because the wife has relied on the economic contribution of the husband to her own economic detriment while she concentrated on homemaking and children, she is entitled to continue to benefit from the husband's career. The law assumes that her contribution to the family has made it possible for him to go to work and enhance his career. Without her he would have had to do both wage earning and homemaking and would have been unable to concentrate on his career. If the wife has not developed her own income-earning capacity because she has stayed home, it would be unfair to now tell her that she must unilaterally absorb the cost of the failed marriage. Today, the needs of the wife, seen in the context of the marital contract, have become the basis for considering alimony.

But the advent of no-fault divorce has not necessarily meant that divorcing people approach divorce from the psychological perspective of no-fault. When one of the couple believes that the other has "caused" the divorce, it is not unnatural to believe that the other spouse should also absorb the consequences of his or her "bad behavior." The psychological stance of the noninitiator of the divorce is "You want this and I don't. So you pay the price and leave me alone." "You want to leave me, so go support yourself!" Or, "You want to leave me? Well, you'd better be prepared to support me anyhow!"

Although there are some cases in which women pay alimony to husbands, most alimony cases involve men paying women. Male resentment of alimony will frequently require discussion by the therapist, either to help the man accept paying it or to help the woman be patient with her husband's resistance. The therapist may want to remind each that the goal of a good divorce is for both husband and wife to feel that economic justice has been done and that both must be able to live decently if future cooperation is to be achieved.

2. *"If she can work, doesn't she have to do so?"* Generally, the wife has an obligation to contribute to her support if she is able. If she has been employed throughout the marriage, she is expected to continue her employment, and her income is applied to meet her needs before alimony is considered. The issue is more complex when she has not been employed throughout the marriage, if she gave up a career to devote herself to home and children, or if she has been employed only part-time because she is caring for children at home.

It is typical for the wife to seek to keep things the same. If the parties mutually decided that she should stay home, it is not surprising that she wants to continue this arrangement. If she has been a homemaker for 25 years and the kids are grown she may be reluctant, and perhaps frightened, to start a career in her late 40s or 50s. Depending on the income of the family, the court may not require her to return to employment. Three factors may influence this decision.

- *Available income.* Is there enough income that the two can maintain the status quo, more or less, without the wife's resuming employment? If the husband earns $65,000 a year as a teacher, and the family has been struggling for years to make ends meet, it will be necessary for her to contribute financially. But if he earns $165,000 as an executive and the two have not been struggling, there will be less pressure on her to begin a career.
- *The wife's earning capacity.* How much can the wife earn? If she has a high school education and can earn $7 an hour, her contri-

bution would be less significant than if she has an MBA and within a year can earn $50,000.

- *The age and needs of the children.* If the wife has been the primary caretaker for the kids and the cost of daycare and after-school supervision would eat up most of her earnings, there is a less compelling argument for her returning to employment than if the youngest child is 16 and can be self-sufficient after school.

All these are issues of need and capacity. The obligation to support is derivative of the implicit marital contracts by which the couple has lived and the pragmatic realities of their finances.

3. *"Why does it have to go on for so long? Don't I have a right to a life too?"* The duration of alimony is generally determined by the length of the marriage and whether it is realistic to expect the wife will earn enough to support herself at an acceptable level. All states provide that alimony ends upon the remarriage of the wife. We know that the majority of divorced women remarry within 10 years.[1] This suggests that a majority of men who are paying alimony will not have to pay it for more than 10 years. On a statistical basis, there is only a one in five chance that a man will have to pay alimony for longer than 10 years. So, what we are discussing when we talk about "long-term or permanent" alimony is helping the male client to manage the risk that his wife will not be married or will not be able to support herself within 10 years. Of course, there is a chance she may never remarry, and the therapist needs to help the male client accept this too and handle his anger.

4. *"How much of my income is she entitled to?"* I have used the phrase "in the style to which she has become accustomed" on several occasions. But this is not an unqualified rule. First is the question whether the couple can afford it. In American society there is no consensus on what people need. Some believe that a 2,000-square-foot house in a middle-class suburb is wonderful; others regard their 6,000-square-foot house as not grand enough. Most people are happy with a Chevrolet or Toyota, but others feel deprived if they can't drive a luxury car. So, what do we really need? The elaboration of need has been so extreme—particularly during the past 15 years—that, once we get beyond basics,

[1]Bramlett, M. D., & Mosher, W. D. (2001). *First marriage dissolution, divorce, and remarriage: United States.* Advance data from Vital and Health Statistics, No. 323. Hyattsville, MD: National Center for Health Statistics.

"need" becomes almost totally subjective. Alimony is supposed to address the subject of need, but we have no legislated or judicial consensus on what people need.

So, we again revert to history and contract. What we "need" is defined by what we are used to. If we have to manage with less than we are accustomed to, we define that as deprivation. So, we tend to equate the status quo with need, even if on a relative basis it seems like extreme luxury to others. The legal notion of "the style to which she is accustomed" is nothing more than a stated preference for the status quo. If two people have lived a frugal existence, this is not the time to ramp up to luxury. And if the two people have had an elaborate lifestyle, the legal system will strip it away only very reluctantly.

If historical lifestyle is an important factor in alimony negotiations, how long must the couple be married for the wife to be entitled to continue in that lifestyle? There is no clear answer. Suppose that Harry was already a millionaire when he married Amber, a nurse with few assets. And suppose they had lived together in his mansion and that he had provided her with a fancy car and a luxurious way of life with fancy vacations, four-star restaurants, and shopping trips at elite stores. Suppose also that she had stopped working as a nurse to devote herself to being Harry's companion. Finally, suppose that they have no children. How long does the marriage have to last for Amber to acquire the right to continuity of lifestyle if they divorce? Few would argue that Amber would have acquired much of an entitlement to alimony after only a 2-year marriage. But what if the marriage lasts 7 years? What about 15 years? The longer the marriage lasts and the more Amber becomes accustomed to this way of life, the greater her claim. And if Amber has given up her career and become rusty in her professional skills, what is Harry's responsibility to compensate for the loss of her career? In medicine the knowledge base changes rapidly. Someone out of nursing for 15 years has missed much of the revolution in computerized records as well as advances in medication and has missed great changes in medical technique. She may be able to requalify as a nurse after a year of study but will now have to compete with others many years her junior. She has lost her seniority and forfeited many years of professional advancement. And no matter how many hours she works as a nurse, she can never earn enough to even approximate the standard of living to which she is now accustomed.

The question of fairness is important here. Suppose that the reason for the divorce is that Harry has grown bored and has found a younger woman. Does this mean anything, or is it just Amber's tough luck? Does she have to unilaterally absorb all the change that results from Harry's restlessness, or does she get protected in any way at all? Fault is not the issue. The issue is whether she has relied to her own detriment on Harry's assurance that they would be together permanently. So, again, the questions are: What is her need? How is that need defined historically? What is her capacity to earn? And what is the husband's capacity to earn?

I encourage couples to articulate the implicit contract that has existed between them during their marriage. I suggest they imagine that they are at the beginning of their marriage and are deciding how to allocate responsibility for earning money and domestic duties between them. They do not yet have children. Each is capable of earning a living and developing a career. But they both envision a traditional life with a home and children. The husband wants his wife to bear children. Childbearing and child raising will distract her from her career. She is willing to take time off but is worried that her capacity to earn will decline. She has seen a study that reports that women lose approximately 3% of their income ceiling for each year they are away from careers. She is willing to take a short maternity leave but will have to return to her career shortly after each child is born. In that event she expects that the husband will take an equal role in caring for the children as they come along. He will be equally responsible for doctor visits, school issues, shopping trips, and the myriad tasks associated with raising children and running the house. He will stay home half the days that a child is home sick and will be equally responsible for transporting children to lessons, soccer games, and similar activities. He will arrange with his employer to be home for dinner with the children, and if his need to work shorter hours interferes with his career he will cheerfully accept the consequences. If he does all of these things, his wife will take responsibility for her own economic future. She will not subordinate her career to the family needs, and she will be as able as her husband to put in the hours necessary for promotion and advancement in the corporate and professional world. That is the alimony-free contract. To the extent that the couple deviates from this scenario and the wife becomes dependent on the husband's income for her future, he acquires an obligation to share the economic risk if the marriage proves unsuccessful, because it would be unfair simply to shift all that risk to her.

I understand that it may be difficult to reconstruct the past as a hypothetical, but it is a useful exercise to cut through the fog of resentment when husbands are asked to part with a significant chunk of future income to support an ex-wife. There has to be some commitment on his part to justice, for without that commitment the divorce will play out as a battle of wills in a courtroom.

THE THERAPIST'S ROLE IN SUPPORT DISCUSSIONS

Once we get to topics relating to money in divorce, the therapist is more likely to be intimidated by the client's statement that "my lawyer said it should be this way." But, notwithstanding the technical aspects of child support and alimony, the discussion raises major emotional issues of entitlement, blame, guilt, fear, dependency, and loss. In materialistic cultures such as ours, it is often difficult to separate identity from consumption, and support issues go right to the heart of identity. It is important that your fear of stepping on lawyers' toes and your discomfort with the arithmetic calculations not intimidate you into abandoning the client to the not very tender mercies of the legal system. Support is an emotional issue, and the therapist needs to stay aware and involved as the client struggles through the issue.

So, what should you do when your client insists that the law in your state allows him to cut off his wife from support because she had an affair? Can you advise him not to, even though you are contradicting his lawyer? Of course you can. It is your job to point out the emotional consequences of legal choices. If alimony is necessary to assure that the wife can succeed in her new life, it should be paid without respect to issues of marital fault–that as we have discussed before–are seldom very clear.

There are a few principles that I present to clients to help avoid angry alimony discussions.

1. Alimony is based on the capacity to pay and the need to receive. It should be mostly an economic decision designed to finance the success of the entire family.

2. The receiving spouse should do whatever he or she can do to generate income. If a woman has young children and is genuinely needed in the home for a period of years by mutual agreement, she

should not have to be employed. But when there are older children who need less care, employment should be a premise if it is at all feasible.

3. The amount of alimony should be sufficient to achieve reasonable parity between the households, particularly when there are children. Economic fairness should apply to the entire family, and no one in the family, including the children, should live at a significantly higher standard than any other.

There is no reason that the therapist cannot have these discussions with either or both spouses even though the therapist may disagree with the advice of the lawyer. It does not constitute the unauthorized practice of law for you to discuss legal issues in the course of advising clients on mental health issues.

Some Principles for Thinking about Alimony

- The longer the marriage lasts, the greater the premise of parity in income.
- Both parties are obligated to contribute, but there has to be recognition of the negative impact of domestic duties on income-producing capacity.
- There is economic value in staying home to attend to children. This applies to both the past and the future.
- In a long-term marriage both partners have acquired the right to maintain the status quo if they can afford it and to share in economic retrenchment if they cannot afford the status quo.
- Alimony is a pragmatic solution to a practical problem. It is not an appropriate vehicle of retribution or vindication.

---

11 Dividing Marital Property

The division of marital property can be a psychologically difficult process, and the client's emotional attachment to particular assets can shape the legal process in potentially destructive ways. Dividing the property can go directly to the heart of the struggles that have destroyed the relationship. Issues of sharing, power, who contributed what value to the marriage, equality or its absence, and entitlement are all powerful emotional questions that can be triggered by the discussion of property. If the husband has long denigrated the wife's contribution to the marriage and now argues that he should get more than half the assets because he produced more, the negotiation of the property division becomes a reprise of his earlier complaints and can become a mutual struggle for vindication rather than a simple division of assets. If the husband has, during the marriage, refused to share financial information with the wife, her fear of hidden assets can cause protracted discovery and financial investigation, which in turn induces acute indignation in the husband. If the wife has been the bigger provider of the two, her resentment of the husband's failure to provide can be expressed through an assertion that he doesn't "deserve" an equal share. And if one of the spouses brought more assets to the marriage, his or her attempt to recapture that money in the distribution of property can precipitate a resentful resistance with the argument that "you may have brought more assets into the marriage initially, but my contribution since then has been more than yours, and you can't have your original contribution back!" So, this becomes another debate over who contributed more and who is more worthy.

Division of assets also creates emotional distress when it threatens the hold of one of the spouses on some asset that has special symbolic value. The most common example in middle-class divorces is the issue of whether the marital home is to be sold or is to be retained for the benefit of the children. The home may represent all the family savings, and the husband (or wife) sees the equity in the house as his only chance that he will ever again possess a house of his own. Or it may represent the wife's only way to preserve a way of life for herself and for the children. The idea of selling it stimulates acute feelings of guilt, anger, and sadness in her. But the house is not the only emotionally laden asset. I have seen intense struggles over the family boat, weekend houses, antique cars, and numerous other assets, some large and others small.

Struggles over these assets can create serious obstacles to settling the divorce and moving on. Lawyers are singularly unequipped to help clients wrestle with the emotional dimensions of property division. Equitable division law has spawned such a panoply of technical issues, tax issues, and experts' reports that it is easy for lawyers to become absorbed in the technical dimensions and entirely miss the symbolic struggle that may well be key to resolving the case.

It can be extremely helpful for the therapist to follow the evolution of the negotiation and offer to help the client explore the emotional implications of any disagreements over assets. It can also be very helpful to explore the issues from the perspective of the nonclient spouse. This will assist the client in finding mutually acceptable options. But, to do this, the therapist needs a primer in the laws of property distribution. Although discussions of assets, stock options, pensions, and houses and mortgages all seem technical, the emotional power of these topics should not be underestimated. I have seen much protracted litigation that could have been avoided if one or both clients had been better helped to explore their intense feelings about some asset and to be better able to understand those of the spouse. Fruitful negotiation requires that each party understand not just the economic significance of the asset but also the emotional and symbolic impact on the other spouse. Again, it may be a struggle, but the therapist should stay engaged with the client even on these complex topics. This chapter is intended to provide both the legal and the emotional basics.

CASE STUDY: MARK AND MARY

Mark and Mary are trying to negotiate how they are going to divide their property, and both are getting angrier by the minute. They married 22 years ago and have two children. Mark is a captain in the local fire department and has only 2 years to go before he is eligible for a pension. The couple has owned a house for 18 years, which is now worth $250,000, with only a $57,000 mortgage balance left. They bought the house in 1985, using a $35,000 inheritance Mary had from her grandmother as their down payment, but they own it jointly. They also have a 401K plan for Mark with $82,000; an IRA of Mary's with $40,000, and some savings bonds inherited by Mark from his mother valued at $28,000. Mark has an antique motorboat he owned before the marriage but restored during the marriage. He estimates it is worth $20,000. Finally, Mary has written and published two cookbooks during the marriage, and last year she received royalties of $6,000 from her publisher.

Mary and Mark have each been to see their respective lawyers in anticipation of discussing property division. Mary's lawyer told her that she was entitled to half of Mark's pension, half of his 401K plan and half of the house plus repayment of the down payment that came from her grandmother's estate. She tells Mark that, although she doesn't seek half of his savings bonds because they were inherited, she wants half of the value of his motorboat. She also says that she feels he is not entitled to any part of the value of her books because she wrote them without any help from him and, in fact, in the face of his discouragement.

As Mary speaks, Mark becomes red with anger.

> "You are so selfish. I've slaved over this house for years. I paid the mortgage, built the deck, repainted the house, rehabilitated the garage and probably doubled its value with my hard work while you did next to nothing. Where do you get off saying that you want the down payment back? That house should be more than half mine, and there is no way you are getting more than half. You want your books because you wrote them, but you want half my pension. What in hell did you do to earn that pension? I worked nights, risked my life, and put up with years of crap from that department so I could retire early. You are not getting half my pension, and I'll see you in court first. You're also not getting the boat. I owned it before we got married, and I slaved to fix it up. It's mine, and you can just forget about it!"

COMMENTARY: Mark and Mary have some serious negotiating to do if they are going to reach agreement. The division of marital property can be complicated. The law is often complex, and some assets can become symbolic for the struggles that stressed the marriage. Eventually, we will watch as Mark and Mary work it out, but first let us review the law of equitable distribution.

OVERVIEW OF EQUITABLE DISTRIBUTION

A hundred years ago most states used a "title" system to distribute property between husband and wife. But, because men owned most of the property, the title method was very unfair to women. In most states courts had no authority to order property transferred from one person to another. The person who had title, whose name was on the property, kept it. Men owned most of the property, because men were the primary economic actors in the family. Most real estate was titled in the husband's name, as was most of the family wealth. So, in a divorce the wife's only hope of financial security was alimony, which was paid only until she remarried or her ex-husband died. And if the court found that the wife's bad behavior was the basis of the divorce–if she was at fault–she could receive no alimony and no property. By today's standards, it was a cruel system.

As a reform, a few states developed the concept of community property. Property acquired during the marriage was assumed to be joint or community property and divided equally upon divorce. But community property was never a popular idea, and some reformers saw it as leading to injustice by permitting wives to get too much property that they did not deserve. The concept of fault and "just desserts" was a persistent theme.

The advent of no-fault divorce called for change in the way property was distributed in divorce. Rules that automatically gave the property to the titled owner became viewed as unjust and discriminatory against women, and because no-fault divorce was itself a reflection of the growing power of women, reform in the laws that governed property division was a logical consequence. So, most states have adopted principles of "equitable distribution" over the last half-century.

Equitable distribution is notable for what it is *not*. The law of equitable distribution empowers courts to transfer property that is defined as "marital" from one spouse to another even though title is only in one name. Having title to the property no longer means that the titled spouse automatically keeps it or that it is not shared with the other spouse. On the other hand, equitable distribution does not mean that the property is equally divided, as it is in community property states. There is no assumption in the law that the property is divided equally between the spouses. So, if it doesn't belong to the person who has title and it isn't automatically divided equally, how is it supposed to be divided?

There is in equitable distribution a complex hodgepodge of principles that the judge is directed to apply. Although these principles are seldom applied in practice, it is instructive to review them briefly. First, marriage is assumed to be an economic partnership. If it dissolves, each partner should be able to take that property that he or she has produced. So, if I created it, I ought to get it. If we created it together, it should be divided between us. But if you had nothing to do with creating it, you should not share in it. If this is the only principle applied, how would Mark and Mary fare in their divorce? Mary did not help earn Mark's pension, and Mark played no direct role in writing her books. Shouldn't each keep the assets that he or she produced?

Equitable distribution law assumes that the contributions of each spouse to any one asset are not easy to distinguish. So, the law requires that the court, when deciding how to distribute the assets, consider the noneconomic contribution of the other spouse. So, the court assumes that a woman who stays home to manage the household and take care of the children made it possible for her husband to keep a job, earn money, and accumulate wealth. So, even though Mary stayed home and Mark was employed as a fireman, it is assumed that her choice to manage the home *made it possible* for him to work, and by doing so she has earned a share of his pension. And his support of her while she wrote her books should entitle him to a share of the book royalties. But that does not necessarily mean that the asset should be divided equally between the two.

Having determined that an asset is marital property (we'll discuss that soon), the court is supposed to apply several other criteria to reach an equitable distribution. It is important to note that the concept of fault is not found among these criteria and is applied only under the most egregious circumstances, such as a case in which a man tried to have his wife murdered. But as a rule, division of property is no-fault.

But now you ask, "With all these criteria, how do we know what a judge would order in any particular case? And if almost all divorces are settled by negotiation and a judge never decides the case, how do we know how to apply these principles?" Before we try to answer these questions, let's look at several other aspects of equitable distribution.

The three stages of equitable distribution are, first, identify marital assets; second, value the assets; and, third, distribute the assets. First, we need to distinguish those assets that are marital and thus subject to equitable distribution.

SEPARATE PROPERTY

Any property owned by one of the partners before the marriage and still owned in the same form is separate property. It belongs to that person alone, and the judge cannot give any part of it to the other spouse. So, an expensive watch Mark owned before the marriage and that he still has remains his. Any property given by a third party to him alone as a gift is his separate property. If his Uncle Mike gave him a camera as a present, it is his alone. Finally, any property that was inherited during the marriage belongs exclusively to the spouse who inherited it. If during the marriage, Uncle Mike died, leaving Mark his car in his will, it is Mark's alone.

But most separate property is not as simple as the watch. Mark had an antique boat before the marriage. Had he never restored it, it would still be his alone. But Mark spent many hours and many dollars on restoring the boat during the marriage. It is no longer separate property. If separate property increases in value as a result of *passive market forces*, it is still separate property, and the increase in value is also separate. This applies to real estate, market accounts, stocks, bonds, and other securities as well. If the increase in value results from simple changes in the market and the spouse did nothing to add to the value, it is still his or her separate property. But note the word "passive." If the increase in value is the result of *active forces*—the application of marital energy or resources—then the increase in value is regarded as marital. Generally, any active creation of wealth during the marriage is marital.

Marital property is anything of value created, acquired, or earned during the marriage. From the day of the wedding to the end of the marriage, all earnings are marital property. So, all of Mark's earnings during the marriage and all the employee benefits such as his pension are marital property. If it was acquired during the marriage and it was not by gift or inheritance, it is, with few exceptions, marital. So, in the case of Mark and Mary the pension, his 401K plan, her IRA, and the royalties from the books she wrote are all marital property and subject to equitable distribution.

COMINGLED ASSETS

A complicated problem arises when a separate asset has been mixed with a marital asset. Disputes over these "commingled" assets have sent many lawyers' children to college. Let's begin with Mark's antique boat. A year before he and Mary got married, he bought it for $1,500. It was a ruined boat, didn't run, and had problems throughout the hull and engine. Had he left it sitting in the garage during the past 20 years and had it increased in value to $10,000, it would still be all his. But during the marriage he restored it to like-new condition. He rebuilt the engine. He haunted flea markets to find spare parts. He lovingly repaired the hull, replaced the rotted wood, and gave it many coats of paint. With Mary's help, he reupholstered and completely reconditioned the seats and interior. He spent hundreds of hours and several thousand dollars restoring the boat. In other words, he poured his energy and money into the boat during the marriage. All of the value added by his effort and all the value added by the marital funds he spent on the boat are now marital assets subject to equitable distribution between him and Mary.

The marital home is a similar problem. Mary used $35,000 of money she inherited from her grandmother for the down payment on the home. Over the years, Mark made the mortgage payments and fixed up the house. The house was purchased in their names jointly, and both signed a large promissory note when they mortgaged the house. Signing a promissory note and incurring debt is the same as investing one's savings. The house is clearly a marital asset. Whether a judge, after a trial, might "trace" Mary's inheritance through the down payment and restore it to her before the rest is divided, one can only speculate. The judge does not have to do so. All of the equity in that house is marital property.

TYPES OF PROPERTY

Property is anything you own that is of value now or in the future. When we think of property, we usually think of tangible assets such as real estate, bank accounts, brokerage accounts, jewelry, and other objects such as cars, boats, or tools. But property includes much more. The divorce process sometimes stretches the definition of "property" beyond what we conventionally regard as property.

The most complicated types of property in divorce are those that have an intangible, future value. One example is anything in the category of intellectual property. Suppose that Mark had spent some of his evenings working in his shop inventing a super-widget and had finally succeeded in obtaining a patent. Even though we have no way of knowing whether there will ever be a market for the device, the patent is marital property, and any money that it might earn in the future is also marital property. The books that Mary wrote are another example. They may or may not sell in the future. But the possibility that they may have future value and generate a stream of cash in the future makes her copyright and royalty agreement with her publisher a marital asset.

Stock options are another category of intangible property. Employees are offered the right to purchase shares of their employers' stock at a preset price called the "strike price," which usually is the price the stock is trading at on the day the option is issued. It has no value that day, because buying at the strike price would not result in a profit. But if the stock price increases, buying at the strike price can produce a significant profit. When the stock market was very robust during the 1990s, many people made fortunes exercising the options their employers had granted. Nowadays, stock options may be less exciting but are nevertheless subject to equitable distribution.

All rights to receive income in the future acquired during the marriage may be marital property. In some states, a professional license or a professional degree may be regarded as marital property even though such property cannot be sold or transferred. It may be the subject of an appraisal, and the value imputed to the license may influence the distribution of other assets. Economics in divorce is not always the same as economics in the real world. Another example is the right to sue someone for damages. If Mark is injured in an accident and loses time from work, he might sue the party responsible for injuring him for damages, such as medical expenses and lost wages. He might also seek compensation for pain and suffering. His lawsuit is marital property. If he wins or settles his suit, some or all of the award may be regarded as marital. Most states treat recovery for pain and suffering as separate property but treat any recovery of economic damages as marital.

An asset that generates high professional fees in divorce is a family-owned business or professional practice. If a man owns a dry cleaning establishment acquired during the marriage, a business appraiser would be hired to determine the value of the business. Because such businesses are bought and sold, determining its value is not complicated. But if a person has a law practice, in which his or her greatest asset is his or her own reputation, the problem of valuation is more difficult. Many states do not permit lawyers to sell their practices. But most states will treat the law practice as a going business on the premise that it would be unfair to the other spouse to disregard it.

Business valuation concerns two parts of a business. The first part is the tangible assets such as fixtures, inventory, machinery, equipment, furnishings, and money owed to the business by its customers (accounts receivable). These "hard" assets are simple to value and present no controversy. The second part of a business is "goodwill," is the intangible part of a business that is essentially the reputation that keeps clients and customers coming back. Without goodwill no business can succeed. In a commercial establishment such as a dry cleaners or a manufacturing firm there are broadly accepted principles for valuing goodwill that reflect the real market value of the business. But the valuation of goodwill in a personal services business or in a professional practice is much harder to understand and often makes clients furious when they first learn about it.

Suppose Marilynn has a law practice in which she earns $350,000 a year. And suppose that she has worked 80-hour weeks for 20 years to build the practice. Also suppose that if she closed her practice and went to work for a large firm her salary would be $200,000. In the jargon of divorce law, Marilynn's entrepreneurial income of $350,000 exceeds her salary income by $150,000. Equitable distribution valuation would assume that this "excess income" is the measure of goodwill of her practice. That excess income would be subjected to a "capitalization ratio" to determine the value of this cash stream. Typically, the capitalization ratio is between one and five times excess earnings, depending on the methodology of the appraiser. So, if the appraiser hired to appraise the value of Marilynn's law practice chose a "cap" ratio of three, he (or she) would value the goodwill of the practice at $450,000. He would also add the value of the hard assets to get a total value of the practice. This is a routine occurrence whenever a spouse has his or her own professional practice. It can generate large professional fees and, occasionally, great bitterness. In conventional adversarial divorce, it is not uncommon for each lawyer to hire an appraiser and for each appraiser to produce a valuation grossly distorted in the direction of the paying client's interest. I recently mediated a case in which the physician husband's accountant valued his medical practice at $200,000 and the wife's accountant valued the same practice at over $2,000,000. Each appraiser had adopted those methodological assumptions that would influence the result in the desired direction. That there are unscrupulous professionals earning a living in the divorce industry is no secret. The challenge for your clients will be to find a neutral expert who will give an objective and honest opinion of value.

NORMS FOR DISTRIBUTION

After assets have been identified and valued, they must be distributed. Here are two hypothetical scenarios to help you understand distribution.

Case Study: Zack and Lisa

Zack and Lisa are in the midst of their divorce and are beginning to wrestle with issues of equitable distribution. In particular, they are having difficulty agreeing on the distribution of the value of Zack's accounting practice. Zack is a successful CPA who worked while earning his bachelor's and master's degrees. Although the couple was married when he was attending school, Zack had maintained a part-time job throughout school and with the help of some student loans had managed to support the family. Lisa had become pregnant during Zack's first year of graduate study and had given up her teaching job when their daughter was born. By the time Zack had graduated and passed the CPA exam, their daughter was 3 years old and attending nursery school. As soon as he was licensed, Zack opened his own practice and quickly became successful.

The couple agreed on a forensic accountant to appraise the practice, and the accountant has submitted a report in which he placed a value of $350,000 on Zack's practice. The couple owns a house that has been appraised at $450,000 and that has an outstanding mortgage balance of $100,000. Lisa has told Zack that she is willing to swap the house for the practice with her receiving the house and Zack retaining his practice.

Scenario 1

When Zack opened his practice, Lisa devoted herself to helping him succeed. To keep his overhead down he brought all his secretarial work and bookkeeping home each night, and she got it done the next day while their child was in nursery school. When he set up the office, she furnished the office with stylish furnishings she found at the lowest price. She spent many hours encouraging Zack when he became discouraged because business had been slow that week. She also entertained frequently so that he could invite potential business contacts to dinner. Throughout the early years of his practice, she was his ever attentive partner in every way. It was only after Zack had been in practice for 5 years that Lisa was able to reduce her involvement. By then, Zack was earning enough to afford a full-time staff and also take enough income to live comfortably. But even then, Lisa continued to serve as his sounding board and to entertain clients. He always credited her with much of his success. "I could never have done it without Lisa," he would tell their friends.

Scenario 2

When Zack started his practice, Lisa was also trying to launch her own career as an artist. She had been an art major in college and had always wanted to become a serious painter. So, she told Zack that although she was supportive of his career, it would be unfair to expect her to do his secretarial work at the price of her own dreams and aspirations. To save money, Zack would stay up late doing his own clerical work. Because Lisa had no interest in cooking or entertaining, he could only entertain clients by taking them out to restaurants. That was very expensive. His wife seldom went along, because she found his clients boring. And because she was so absorbed in her painting, she really did not take any interest when he wanted to talk about the problems at work. Now, 10 years later, Zack felt that his success as an accountant was due entirely to his own efforts. In the meantime, Lisa had filled their attic with completed paintings but, with the exception of the few paintings bought by sympathetic friends and relatives, had sold almost nothing.

COMMENTARY: If we are looking at Scenario 1, the division of the assets is probably quite simple, Lisa was a full-life partner in the creation of Zack's practice, and her suggestion of trading the house for the practice does not cause a problem for Zack.

When Zack consults his attorney, he is told that because Lisa's contribution to his practice was substantial she is entitled to a substantial share. The lawyer quotes the law of equitable distribution that cites the contribution of each partner to the economic value of the assets. So, Zack agrees to Lisa's suggestion. The house and the practice have approximately the same value, and he regards each of them as entitled to half. The case settles easily.

The problem arises in Scenario 2.

Clearly, Lisa was no help to Zack. She let him struggle while she pursued her own unproductive career. Although Zack had tolerated Lisa's "career," he had always felt that she was being self-indulgent in staying with it long after it was evident to everyone else that she lacked the talent or the knack for commercial success. He also resented how Lisa spent her time and the money that he earned. When Lisa wasn't painting, she was often at the gym or on the tennis court. As soon as he had started to generate a good income, she had hired a housekeeper to manage the domestic chores and justified it by saying it was necessary to her career. In Zack's estimation, Lisa was spoiled and lazy and had spent 10 years "playing" at his expense. The idea that she would claim half the value of the practice he had created without help from her was infuriating. And her blithe insistence that he pay her alimony in addition was enough to send him into a rage.

When he consults his attorney, he does not get the answers that he wants. His attorney tells him that in the state where they are, there is a presumption that the assets will be split 50/50 between the spouses and that the burden of proof is on the one who says he or she should get more than half. It is true that the law considers who contributed what to the marriage and that if they went to trial and got the right judge, that judge might award him more than half—perhaps as much as two-thirds or even, if they put in a great case, as much as three-quarters. The cost of carrying the litigation all the way to trial would be in the neighborhood of $50,000, according to the lawyer, and Zack, who has witnessed a lot of litigation among his clients, fully understands how quickly the bill can run up.

Sure enough, when Zack and Lisa talk, she tells him that according to her lawyer she is entitled to half of everything. She says that she ran the household for all those years and is entitled to half. And besides, she tells him, if her career had been successful, he would have been entitled to half the value of her paintings. In fact, she is willing to give him half the paintings in the attic; so, in case she becomes successful in the future, he can reap the benefits by selling the paintings. Zack is furious.

COMMENTARY: Zack has a choice in Scenario 2. He can act on his indignation and accept the costs of the struggle, or he can pay Lisa more than he thinks she is entitled to. Let's look at the costs and benefits.

Cost–Benefit Analysis

According to Zack's lawyer, his best-case possibility in court is three-quarters of the practice. Lisa seeks one-half of his practice, or $175,000. If he tries the case–and wins–she gets only one-half of that, or $87,500. If it costs him $50,000 in legal fees, his best-scenario gain is $37,500, which is the difference between what he pays her and what the lawyer charges him. Note that this is his *best-case* outcome. If he tries the case and the judge awards him 60%, he saves $35,000–the difference between 50% and 60%. But, because it will still have cost him $50,000 in legal fees, he will have lost $15,000 even though he "won" on the issue.

But there are also some other downside risks. First, he might not win, in which case he will have wasted $50,000. Second, the judge could direct him to pay Lisa's attorney fees, which could be as high as his–another $50,000. Further, the time it takes to go to trial is time he cannot be earning money. And the anxiety about the struggle will also distract him from his practice. With discovery, depositions, and court appearances, the case could easily consume 200 hours of Zack's time. During that time he might have earned $100,000. So, the total downside risk for Zack if everything goes wrong is closer to $200,000, just to take a chance at saving $37,500. If this were analyzed as a business risk, it would be a bad deal.

On a strictly economic basis, it makes more sense for Zack to agree to Lisa's demand for half than it makes to fight her for three-quarters. But for some people, that is a hard proposition to swallow. Like many men, Zack is very likely to get swept up in "the principle of the thing." Why should she get something she isn't entitled to? Why should she be allowed to use the system to extort money from me? Am I a wimp or what? I can't just roll over. What kind of man am I? Lawyers love this reasoning, because it guarantees large legal fees. But it is still makes no sense in the final analysis.

Lisa has also been advised by her lawyer that she could lose at trial. The judge could find that her contribution to the marriage did not earn her half of Zack's practice. And the judge could refuse to order Zack to pay her legal fees. So, Lisa has her own cost–benefit problem. She wants to start life as a single woman. She does not want the divorce hanging over her for another year or two. And she doesn't want the divorce to be bitter, because she knows that would be bad for the children. So, she has considerable motivation to negotiate and compromise. Were Zack to offer her 45% of the value of his practice, she could live with it. It would give him a symbolic victory, and he might go away feeling vindicated. For Zack, another 5% of his practice is worth $17,500 in his pocket at no cost. If your client is in this situation, encourage him or her to think in terms of symbolic resolution and dollars-and-cents arithmetic. Saving legal fees and time that could otherwise be used for earning money, building a career, or sending the kids to college is far more valuable than fighting over assets and their valuation. In the long run, litigation in this type of situation is a sure loser. Although some lawyers might help their clients reach the wise decision not to litigate this case, many others would not. Although the therapist might find the arithmetic here daunting, there is nothing so complicated that you could not at least direct the client to an accountant who could help with the numbers. Once again, this is a choice between acting on one's feelings or acting in one's interest. The therapist is superbly situated to encourage this type of evaluation.

THE POWER OF 50/50

Even though equitable distribution laws have been designed to calibrate justice better than crude 50/50 formulas, the legal profession has nevertheless defaulted to 50/50. Lawyers don't get sued for malpractice when settling for half the assets. To fully apply the law and come to agreement on all the factors that the judge is admonished to consider is an intellectual task worthy of a Talmudic scholar. If your client has an unlimited budget and unlimited time and the good fortune to draw a smart judge who is not overloaded with work, the law may be applied in all its subtle elegance. But warn your client not to count on it.

I remember when I was a child sitting with my brother watching my mother cut a piece of cake into two equal parts. Even a few millimeters difference in the size of the two pieces was enough to provoke a fight between us. In our society, we spend our formative years observing numerous political struggles for equality—among races, religions, sexes, and people with different sexual orientations, to name but a few examples. We learn to regard anything less than half as *unfair.* We are raised to equate fair with equal. And in the absence of very compelling logic to the contrary, we readily default to 50/50. The public might well be much better off if the property distribution laws simply required the distribution of marital property to both parties equally. Perhaps such a crude standard might result in an occasional injustice. But in the long run it would save divorcing people millions of dollars in legal fees. Think about the logic of the demand for more than half the assets. When a husband, for example, proposes that he deserves more, he is also proposing that she deserves less. It takes a strong personality not to experience such a suggestion as an attack on her value and self-worth. The statement that "I contributed more than you did" becomes a reprise of the struggles that led to the divorce originally. It is very unlikely that she can accept the proposition. Those are fighting words for sure and are not worth the price that he will pay for them. But how will you convince him of this? In order to do so, you will require an understanding of the psychological factors that complicate a couple's approach to equitable distribution.

THE PSYCHOLOGY OF EQUITABLE DISTRIBUTION

The issue that troubles Zack in our hypothetical case is not the only one that affects the way people feel about equitable distribution. They often are troubled by the belief that their spouses were lazy, or big spenders. This is particularly intense among men, who are usually the noninitiators of the divorce. "I don't want this divorce. I didn't do anything wrong. Why does she get half my property?" It is also an issue when one spouse thinks that their soon-to-be ex-spouse has better economic prospects. The wife may have a more dynamic career. The husband may anticipate a large inheritance. All of these issues can generate a strong belief that justice requires that your client get more than half. But all run up against the same norm of 50/50 division.

For both men and women, the issue is tricky. If, for example, the man wishes his wife to agree to take less than half of a particular asset or to take less than half of all the assets, he will need a more persuasive argument than "I deserve it and you do not." It would be advisable for him to cite her greater prospects, his greater need, or some other reason that does not imply that she deserves less—because, as soon as he introduces that argument, he will be met with stiff resistance by the default position of 50/50. Few lawyers will encourage a client to take less than half without very compelling reasons.

The reverse also happens frequently. One spouse, most often the wife, cites the husband's greater earning capacity as the reason that she should get more than half the assets. If he has already addressed that issue through the discussion of alimony, her argument will not be compelling. But if she is waiving alimony and he has significantly greater income or prospects for much higher income than she has, he may find her argument compelling. In many cases he can concede a little more than half and defuse the issue. Or he may default to 50/50. It is an emotionally powerful position.

THE LINK BETWEEN EQUITABLE DISTRIBUTION AND ALIMONY

In most states, the law of both alimony and equitable distribution instructs the judge to consider one when deciding the other. Alimony is based on need. So, if a wife is receiving millions of dollars in equitable distribution, her ability to generate investment income may be so great that her need for alimony is reduced or eliminated. But only a very small percentage of couples have this level of wealth.

An issue that often arises here is how much income to attribute to the capital received by each spouse. If the wife receives $1,000,000 and we assume that she can earn 6%, then we are assuming investment income of $60,000 annually–but only half of that if we assume a reinvestment rate of 3%. The discussion of imputed income quickly becomes a question of risk. The more aggressively invested, the more income or growth a portfolio will generate in the short run. But the more aggressively invested, the greater the risk of a calamitous decline in the market, with a resulting loss of capital. During the 1990s, when the stock market appeared stuck in a rising mode, people felt comfortable assuming very high rates of return. The Dow Jones Industrial index has averaged growth of 11% a year over the past 40 years. But the stock market collapse of 2000–2002 dashed the optimism that prevailed for so long. So, nowadays it is not unusual to hear the wife's lawyer argue that we can only assume income of 2% or 3% if the portfolio is invested wisely.

When discussing income imputed to investment as it relates to the need for alimony, the issue of savings also arises. Suppose the investment income imputed to the wife's capital is $60,000 a year and she claims a need for $100,000 a year of income. Does that mean that she needs only $40,000 a year in alimony? If the history of the marriage reflects a pattern of annual savings, she will argue that she is not obliged to consume all of the investment income but rather is entitled to let it accrue so that her investment grows each year. So, for example, she may argue that she is entitled to accrue 2% to account for inflation and another 2% to account for growth. This leaves only 2% or $20,000, actually contributed toward her annual need. Ergo, she argues, she should receive an additional $80,000 annually in alimony. This can become very contentious.

Most people do not have enough capital that they have to worry much about investment income. Most middle-class couples have some equity in their house, one or two retirement plans, and maybe less than $100,000 in liquid assets. By the time the assets are divided, each party is worth a few hundred thousand dollars, at best, and imputed investment income is not an issue. In these cases, alimony must be provided from current income—which accounts for the bitter resistance of many who are expected to pay alimony.

Some discussion of men receiving alimony is appropriate here even though it is still an unusual thing. There are an increasing number of two-income couples in which the wife outearns her husband. There are also more couples in which the partners switch traditional roles and the husband stays home and becomes a house-husband. If the wife's income is significantly greater than the husband's, it is not surprising to see a demand that the wife pay alimony to the husband. Notwithstanding the growth of equality for women, most women are shocked when it is suggested that they pay alimony. But courts will award alimony to a man who has been an economically dependent spouse. This may be the source of great anger.

DISCOVERY AND THE MYTH OF HIDDEN ASSETS

We have discussed the Greek chorus phenomenon, in which ill-informed friends and relatives advise people about their divorces and tell them how they are about to get screwed. The suggestion is that the husband must be hiding assets and that only an aggressive lawyer will be able to find them. This particular advice is aimed at the wife. When this advice succeeds in kindling the fears of the wife, the only ones who profit are the lawyers.

The truth is at significant variance with the myth. In very few divorces are hidden assets a problem. Few people are in a position to hide assets successfully. First, it requires a lot of assets to hide. This rules out most people. Second, because little income is received in cash, it is easy to trace most assets through a "paper trail." Those who are in cash businesses, such as restaurant owners, may have access to significant amounts of cash. But in order to hide cash from one's spouse, one must also hide it from the government. Successfully hiding assets requires tax evasion. In my experience, couples routinely taking "hot cash" are both knowledgeable about how much they have taken, and both are aware where the stash is hidden (usually in a safe deposit box). So, the actual incidence of people hiding large amounts of money is infrequent.

This does not necessarily mean that there is not controversy about other economic issues. In cases involving professional practices or small businesses, it is not uncommon for the spouse running the business to argue that business is down and the value of the business is reduced, for purposes of equitable distribution and support discussions. Recent reductions in income give rise to cynicism, and "RAIDS"–or "recently acquired income deficiency"–is a cliché among lawyers. Most of these disputes center on accounting interpretations of expense reporting, in which the spouse operating the business defends the expenses listed as legitimate while the other spouse, typically the wife, argues that expenses have been overstated to distort the true income of the business. These are legitimate issues about which people of goodwill can disagree. But these are not about hidden assets.

HOW TO AVOID THE PROBLEM

The best way to avoid suspicions is not to create them in the first place. Generally, how money is discussed during the divorce reflects how money was managed during the marriage. If a spouse was secretive or duplicitous about money during the marriage, we can expect distrust and suspicion during the divorce. But if the financial dealings were open and honest during the marriage and neither spouse does anything to destroy that trust during the divorce, the couple should be able to avoid suspicion and unnecessary discovery on the part of lawyers. Thus, therapists need to encourage clients to be forthright and honest in disclosure. They also need to serve as a reality check for clients who have exaggerated fears that something is being hidden. If the spouse has been honest in the past, chances are good that he or she is being honest now.

PENSIONS

There are two types of pensions: defined benefit plans and defined contribution plans. A defined contribution plan, such as a 401K plan, is one in which the employee has deposited part of his or her earnings and the employer has deposited some matching amount. There are several variations of the 401K plan, but all are worth whatever is in them. They are defined by what has been contributed plus whatever growth (or loss) has accrued. An individual retirement account (IRA) is also a defined contribution plan. These are accounts that receive tax-deferred income (in the case of standard IRAs) and can earn money that is also not taxed until it is withdrawn, usually after one reaches age 58. If the person withdraws money before this age, the amount withdrawn is subject to taxes and penalties. (Roth IRAs are slightly different, with contributions already taxed and withdrawals not subject to taxation.) Defined contribution plans do not present valuation problems because they are worth whatever the balance is at the time of the distribution.

The type of pension plan that can become a headache is the defined benefits plan. These pension plans have no account balance. They are a contractual right a person has earned through employment. The employer promises to pay the employee a certain amount of money upon retirement, after achieving some particular age. Most defined benefits plans provide a formula that depends on the number of years of employment and the income earned by the employee at the time of retirement. So, for example, a state teachers plan may provide that a teacher can retire at age 65 and after she has completed 20 years of service. In many plans, retirement income is a percentage, for example one-half, of the average annual income earned during the last 3 years of employment. So, if average earnings were $80,000 annually during the last 3 years, the pension would be $40,000 a year.

Pension plans vary considerably, with some more generous than others. Some plans such as police and firemen's plans allow retirement after 20 years of service, regardless of the employee's age. These plans are very valuable because, if one retires at age 40 and has a life expectancy of 85, he or she will collect the pension for 45 years. This could amount to several million dollars by the time of death. Some pensions are indexed for inflation, which means that the amount of the pension will increase each year to keep pace with inflation.

The problem with defined benefit plans in divorce consists in the manner in which they are distributed. There are two ways to distribute them, one of which is easy and one of which is difficult. The easy way is called deferred distribution. The pension is divided when it goes into pay status. Using a document called a qualified domestic relations order, the judge directs the pension plan administrator to sequester a portion of the pension acquired during the marriage and to pay the appropriate portion to the spouse when the employed spouse actually begins to receive it. So, assume a marriage of 10 years between a male police officer who was employed for 5 years before he married. If he is getting divorced, two-thirds of the pension rights he has acquired is regarded as marital, because the portion acquired before the marriage is not marital; whatever rights he acquires after the divorce is also not marital. If he is projected to retire at 20 years of service, one-half of his pension will be subject to distribution. If he and his wife agree to an equal division, she will receive approximately one quarter of his pension check when he begins to collect it. In deferred distribution there are no complex calculations on which the spouses have to agree.

The more difficult form of distribution is called the offset method. A pension is similar to an annuity. An employee can go to an insurance company and tell them that he (or she) wants to buy an annuity that pays $1,000 a month starting at age 60 and continuing until he dies. The company will calculate what that would cost them (assuming that he lives to some actuarially assumed age), calculate projected interest rates, and add a profit. Then they tell him that they will agree to his request if he pays them $80,000. What they have done is to convert the future stream of cash payments to a present value in which they assume that the money he pays them will generate enough income to cover their payments to him as well as earn a profit for them. Any future cash stream can be reduced to a present value.

The difficulty arises when we try to establish the present value of the pension. The calculation of present value is based on a number of actuarial assumptions, including prevailing interest rates, the age at which the employee is assumed to retire, and whether or not the pension is indexed for inflation. Depending on the assumptions made by the actuary, the present value of a particular pension can vary greatly. One actuary might calculate the present value of a pension at $100,000 while another calculates it at $300,000. As with many other expert witnesses that service the divorce industry, actuarial science has its share of whores who tilt their findings in the direction of the client paying the bill. So, one problem is the inconsistency of findings in actuarial reports.

A second problem arises when we try to distribute the assets. Suppose that the pension valuation is $300,000. And suppose that there is a house with equity of $200,000 as well as various savings totaling $100,000. Suppose further that the husband, who is the one with the pension, is 50 years old and will pay alimony and child support. In fact, he cannot retire at 65 because he will not have enough assets to do so. Finally, assume that the couple agrees that all property will be divided equally. If we do an offset in which the husband keeps his pension, the wife must get everything else. Although the husband can look forward to his full pension 15 years hence, he has no access to assets and no savings for those 15 years. It would make much more sense for this couple to do a deferred distribution in which the wife gets her share of the pension when it goes into pay status in 15 years and for the couple to divide the other $300,000 between them. Now they would each have access to $150,000 in capital with which to rebuild their lives.

Offset distribution works only when the present value of the pension is small or when there are a lot of other assets, so that each spouse has some liquid assets as well as retirement assets.

In some cases the pension is a hot emotional issue. Some governmental employees, particularly police and firemen, have pensions that allow them to retire at a young age after putting in 20 years on the job. For a police officer who started in his early 20s this could mean retirement with a significant pension at an early age. He can then begin a second career and enjoy two incomes or can spend the rest of his life in relative leisure. For policemen in particular who have very stressful careers, the promise of early retirement is an important motivation that keeps them employed. But it's a problem in divorce. Because a policeman can retire early and possibly collect his pension for 40 years or more, the present value of these pensions can be enormous, dwarfing all other assets of the couple. Consequently, the offset method of division, in which the cop keeps the entire pension while the spouse gets other assets, doesn't work. So, the pension has to be divided when it goes into pay status. For an officer who was planning to retire in a few years, this can be enraging, because he suddenly finds himself with half the pension he thought he had. For many, it means they must continue in a job they may dislike—because they can no longer afford to get out. For the cop who is not the initiator and who resents the divorce, this can indeed be a bitter pill.

Therapists in this situation will be challenged to help the client manage these feelings without derailing the divorce. Discussion of the goals of good divorce may not be enough, and the client may actually need assistance mourning the loss of a long-held dream. These are difficult cases.

THE MARITAL HOME

Many couples have most of their equity invested in their house. At least one has to move out and establish another household. Consider the typical couple, in which the wife will be the parent of primary residence for the two young children and the children will spend alternate weekends and at least one night during the week with their father. The wife usually wants to stay in the house as long as possible. She is attached to the house—and it is not just a house; it is *home*. Moreover, she worries about the children and believes that the best thing for kids is to have as little disruption as possible. So, she is resistant to any possibility that requires the house to be sold. Whether there are practical options to selling the house depends on many other factors.

First, does the couple have enough income to keep the house? Many couples have bought a more expensive house than they can really afford. In these families we often find that both spouses are employed and that the entire salary of one is dedicated to the mortgage and taxes on the house. If the wife and kids stay in the house, her total costs could claim 80% of family income. There would not be enough income left, after paying support, for the husband to live a middle-class life. Not only do the couple have too little income, but also all their savings are tied up in the house; so, until the equity is liquidated, the husband cannot own a home of his own. He can live with this situation for a year or two, but eventually he will become resentful.

A second question is: What other assets do they have? Ideally, if the wife stays in the house, she should buy out the husband's interest, using other assets. If they have enough assets so that she can keep the house and have at least some cushion of cash, and if the cost to support the house is realistic with reasonable support from the husband, this may work well. She may be willing to live "rent-poor."

The least desirable option is to continue to own the house jointly. It is difficult to agree on managing repairs and maintenance. It keeps both spouses' capital tied up and keeps them tied together economically at a time when they are trying to achieve separate lives. Finally, most such agreements provide that the house will be sold at a future date, typically when the youngest child graduates from high school. So, while this arrangement postpones the inevitable, she will have to move eventually. This often engenders continued resentment on her part. The couple should explore any amicable way to avoid this. They may benefit by reviewing what the house has come to mean symbolically and emotionally to each one. Many people derive part of their identity from the status and appearance of their house–they wear the house like a garment. Clients may need help in letting go of old dreams in order to put new and more practical ones in place.

DEBT

Debt is offset against assets. Just as we subtract the mortgage from the value of the house to determine equity, we also subtract the value of all debts to determine the couple's net worth. Debt acquired during the marriage is marital debt, just as assets acquired during the marriage are marital assets. And, as with assets, it does not matter whose name is on the debt. If it is acquired during the marriage, it is marital. Some debts cause more problems than others. Debt incurred over the objection of one spouse often causes resentment when the other spouse is told that he or she is equally responsible for the debt. Short-term debt often reflects the disarray that accompanies divorce. Couples who are already incurring deficits incur more as they separate and begin supporting two households. So, $10,000 or even $30,000 of credit card debt can accumulate quickly. The problem with credit card debt is that the interest is so ferocious that minimum monthly payments become a large part of the monthly budget. This requires ever more use of credit cards, and the couple gets trapped in a rising level of debt. If that describes your clients, it requires immediate attention before it becomes too big to handle without a bankruptcy.

I counsel people to regard debt with the same pragmatism I encourage throughout the separation. Incurring debt is the same as spending assets. Once money is spent, it is gone. It does not matter that someone should have, would have, or could have done something else, had one been wiser. Debt must be paid off. Short-term debt should be paid off first, because it is so costly. Any liquid assets available should be used for this purpose. If there is still equity in the house, a second mortgage or a refinanced first mortgage may be a solution to paying credit card debt. If modest amounts of short-term debt remain for each spouse to pay off in the future, that is all right–but not more than a few thousand dollars each. And they need agreement that neither will continue to incur further credit card debt. Credit card debt is a measure of disarray, so it is a subject that often reveals underlying emotional agendas. As such, it is another opportunity for the therapist to help clients avoid litigation. Many clients are very angry about debt incurred by the other spouse and sometimes insist that the other spouse take sole responsibility for repaying the debt. The law does not generally support this and treats debt incurred during the marriage as an offset against assets acquired during the marriage. Clients need to be reminded, yet again, that this is not the time or opportunity to vindicate the emotional issues that precipitated the divorce.

DEBT TO PARENTS

Debt to the parents of one of the spouses can also be a problem. For example, suppose the wife's parents loaned the couple $30,000 for the down payment on the house 10 years ago. When they made the loan, they did not specify a repayment date, did not require payment of interest, and simply said to pay it back someday when the couple could afford it. Now, the divorcing wife claims that the two of them have to pay back her parents. The husband believes the money was really a gift and doesn't see why he should have to pay it back after all these years. In some states the absence of a promissory note, a history of interest payments, or other indicator of debt might allow him to escape without repayment. In others, a judge might or might not recognize the debt or might conclude that it was a gift to the couple and is marital property. To take advantage of the situation sows long-term seeds of resentment. It should be obvious that the wife's parents did not intend to make a gift to the husband to be carried away by him after a divorce. If he takes money they believe he is not entitled to, he will destroy the possibility of goodwill from them.

It is a genuine loss, from the perspective of the children. The money, in some way, should revert to their family. This is yet another example of how the vindication of a legal right may not be worth the emotional cost.

One final note about debt. Several times a year I see a couple who, through bad management or financial misfortune, have so much debt that they are strangling in it. They will not be able to pay it off in the foreseeable future and also thrive. Such couples should consider bankruptcy. Bankruptcy, though regarded by many as a stigma, is actually the result of historical reform. It grew as a reform in the days of debtors' prisons. Its purpose is to give people overwhelmed by bad fortune a clean start in life. The husband and the wife each have an absolute right to go bankrupt. If either files for bankruptcy, he or she may be able to discharge all the debt in his or her name, including debt for which both are liable. Or, at the least, he or she will be able to restructure and reduce the debt to manageable proportions. Just because they are married does not mean that each is responsible for the other's debts. If a loan is not in the name of the wife and is only in the name of the husband, if he discharges it in bankruptcy, his creditors cannot seek repayment from his spouse. But if it is a joint debt and only one spouse discharges it, the creditors can seek payment from the other. So, if most of the debts are joint and the couple is overwhelmed by debt, it is important that they declare bankruptcy together. If this is something to consider, they should be referred to a bankruptcy lawyer for consultation. No one likes to think about bankruptcy, but if it means the difference between a family's being able to thrive or not, it should be considered carefully. It is well within the therapist's scope to encourage an overwhelmed couple to explore this alternative.

CUTOFF DATE

Assets acquired during the marriage are subject to equitable distribution. The marriage begins on the day of the wedding, but precisely when it ends may be more complicated. In most states, the cutoff date for equitable distribution is the day when one of the spouses first files for divorce. The cutoff date is significant, because anything acquired after that date is not marital property. So, if the wife buys a lottery ticket and wins the jackpot on the day after the divorce complaint is filed, she is under no obligation to share her winnings with her husband. For most people the cutoff date is not quite so dramatic, because in the few months that it is going to take to get things resolved they are unlikely to receive a big windfall. But there are some routine acquisitions that may be affected. If the husband's employer makes contributions to his pension plan on a routine basis, the contributions that occur after the cutoff date are his alone. If he gets a bonus after that date, it may be all his. If the bonus includes a rewards for work performed before the cutoff date, that portion of the compensation will be regarded as marital. But if the cutoff date was a year ago and he gets a bonus for work done only since that date, then it is his alone.

The date the divorce complaint is filed is an absolute cutoff date. Most states provide that the cutoff date is regarded as the day the marriage ended. However, this can be difficult to establish. If a wife tells her husband that she wants a divorce on January 1, it could be claimed that that is the day the marriage ended. But if he convinces her to try marital counseling and they try that for 3 months unsuccessfully, when did the marriage end? Certainly the date of separation is a good indicator. But what happens if they continue to have sex after they have separated? Is the marriage truly at an end upon the separation? The issue can be rancorous if one spouse wants to establish an earlier date than the other because to do gives him or her an advantage. If they have decided to mediate, they will probably conclude negotiations in a few months, during which time it is unlikely to matter. But if they contemplate a long process or long period of separation before signing a separation agreement, they should agree on a cutoff day and memorialize it in a memo signed by both.

PREPARING TO NEGOTIATE

In preparation for negotiation, both spouses should develop proposals. Each proposal should include the reasoning behind the proposed division of each asset. The result should be a table showing all assets and liabilities that would belong to each, were they to agree to the proposal.

Let's return to Mark and Mary, whom we met at the beginning of the chapter. Mark has prepared a table showing his proposed distribution of assets between him and Mary:

Asset	Value	Mary	Mark
House equity	$193,000	$193,000	
Mary's IRA	$40,000	$40,000	
Projected value of Mary's book royalties	$30,000	$30,000	
Antique boat	$20,000		$20,000
Mark's pension	$350,000		$350,000
Mark's savings bonds (exempt), *not included in total*	$28,000		
Mark's 401K	$82,000	$82,000	
Joint savings account	$16,000		$16,000
Mary's 2004 Jeep	$18,000	$18,000	
Mark's 2000 Honda	$4,000		$4,000
Household furnishings	$30,000	$30,000	
Totals	$783,000	$393,000	$390,000

Mary reviewed Mark's proposal with her lawyer. He told her that at trial she would probably get half of everything but that much of Mark's argument had merit. A perfect 50/50 division would have each of them getting $391,500 at face value, slightly less than she gets under Mark's proposal. With the tax benefits she was getting in the house she probably had at least half of the net tax value already. Mary thought about it and agreed.

COMMENTARY: Mark has made a reasoned proposal in which he has taken both his own and Mary's interests into account, and it has been accepted. Mary might have held out for a few more dollars, and Mark probably would have conceded. But the way this developed was quite realistic. For a small percentage of divorcing couples the division of assets may be more complicated than that of this couple. But for most, the division will be close to 50/50 and will not be the most difficult issue.

CONCLUSION

Asset division can be surprisingly difficult for some people. Even though equal division is typical, disputes over relatively small amounts of money can be intense, because these items have come to symbolize the issues that broke up the marriage. Property issues can touch issues of entitlement, vindication, sharing, and many other hot emotions. The therapist can be kept busy helping clients to sort out the feelings from the real economic issues so that small economic issues do not derail the negotiation about the major issues.

12 Helping Clients Manage the Economic Challenges of Divorce

In the preceding chapter I provided an overview of the law of equitable distribution as well as the support issues of alimony and child support. In this chapter we explore how these subjects are involved in some of the most intense emotional struggles of divorce. Certainly, struggles over money and property occupy far more time and energy than struggles over children. And conflict over economic issues can leave divorcing couples as bitter and disorganized as the most poisonous custody fight.

CASE STUDY: MAX AND SARA

Max and Sara have been married for 20 years and live in a northeastern suburb. They have three children, ages 9, 13, and 16. Max is employed as a mortgage broker and earns an average of $80,000 a year in commissions. His income, as with all commission-based income, fluctuates and is influenced by the state of the real estate market and shifts in interest rates. Max is 50 years old. Sara has not been employed for the past 14 years. She worked as a computer analyst until she became pregnant with the couple's second child and has been a full-time homemaker ever since. When she was employed, she earned $50,000 a year in a senior position. But having been out of her career for so long, she believes that her skills now are so obsolete that she would literally have to start from the beginning. Besides, at age 49 and with three demanding children to raise, she has no desire to return to work.

Although Max and Sara have always tried to be frugal, the pressure of having three children has always consumed just about everything they earned. They live in a house that they bought 6 years ago for $245,000 and which is now worth about $300,000. They have a mortgage of $180,000 and monthly costs for mortgage payments and real estate taxes are $1,750 per month. They have little savings–a few thousand dollars–other than some IRAs worth about $20,000 and Max's 401K retirement plan, worth about $140,000. They have had some heavy dental bills for their kids recently as well as some expensive repairs to the house that have run up their home equity loan and some credit card debts. The home equity loan is for $25,000, and the credit card debt is at $12,000. From an economic standpoint, Max and Sara are an unremarkable middle-class couple.

The couple is now talking divorce after Sara told Max that she wanted to end the marriage. They have been through several rounds of marriage counseling in an attempt to deal with a relationship that has cooled and grown more distant over the years. Like so many women in contemporary America, Sara has decided that the lack of intimacy and the vacuum of communication between her and Max is simply intolerable. She believes that, as painful as the divorce will be, she can't go on living this unsatisfying and emotionally empty existence. Max, who acknowledges that Sara is unhappy, nevertheless believes that the two of them should stay together and work at it for the sake of the family. But Sara is adamant, and the couple is now trying to figure out how to manage the divorce.

COMMENTARY: The economic realities for Max and Sara are daunting. Max has take-home pay that averages $6,500 per month. The current monthly budget for the family is itemized in Sidebar 12.1. It is immediately evident that the total monthly budget slightly exceeds what Max brings home in a good year. Max is always nervous that a few bad months will leave him unable to pay the bills on the first of the month. And when there is an extraordinary expense for a major repair, a school trip, or a couple of root canals, the answer is always to put it on the credit card or increase the home equity loan. If the couple just barely squeaks by in one household, how are they going to be able to afford two households? We know that if Max moves out, as Sara wants him to do, it will only reduce the cost of this household by about 15% at most, or about $1,000. But no court would oblige Max to pay 85% of his income as support

Sidebar 12.1. Max and Sara's Current Monthly Expenses Prior to Their Decision to Separate

Mortgage and taxes	$1,750
Home equity loan	$250
Homeowners insurance	$90
Heat and utilities	$220
Phone	$90
Cell phones	$100
Cable TV	$80
Routine repairs	$100
Total housing	$2,590
Car payment–Sara	$325
Leased car–Max	$405
Auto insurance	$180
Maintenance	$100
Gasoline	$200
Total automotive	$1,210
Food and sundries	$750
Restaurants	$200
Prescription drugs	$80
Newspapers and magazines	$40
Clothing	$350
Hair care	$75
Life insurance	$100
Psychotherapy	$200
Unreimbursed medical	$80
Unreimbursed dental	$100
Credit card payment	$350
Children's lessons	$100
Summer camp	$120
Vacation fund	$300
Total personal expenses	$2,795
Total monthly budget	$6,595

for the family. So, if we assume that Max's departure would leave Sara and the children in the house with a monthly budget of $5,600, his obligation for alimony and child support would be about half or slightly more than half of his income. Even if we assume that Max is generous and pays 60% of his income for support, Sara would have $3,900 available to support a budget of $5,600.

This does not include additional expenses, such as lawn care and yard work that Max does himself. Unless Max continues these chores, or unless Sara and the children take over that job, it would add about $250 a month to the cost. Moreover, the couples' oldest child is about to get her driver's license, which will add about $100 per month to the household auto insurance. Finally, there is absolutely no allowance here for any savings for college or for retirement other than Max's 401K plan, and it is unlikely that he will be able to continue to contribute.

DIVORCE AND ECONOMIC CHANGE

A continuing theme of this book is that divorce requires change on the part of all family members. The only question is how that change will be distributed across the family. Will change be distributed fairly, or will it be piled on one member in order to avoid change for others? It is completely evident that the family cannot reorganize into two households without major economic changes. Here are the choices:

1. A 30–40% reduction in living standards across the board appears unavoidable. This requires the elimination of all discretionary spending and a significant reduction in spending in many areas regarded as necessary. Sidebar 12.2 itemizes the reductions that might get Sara and the kids close to a budget of $3,900 per month, despite a persistent deficit of $450/month.
2. The couple temporarily can draw upon their limited savings to finance their deficit. But they will exhaust all their savings within a few years.
3. Alternatively, they can increase income by having Sara return to work. This may or may not solve the problem, depending on how much Sara will earn.

Sidebar 12.2. Expenses Sara Has to Reduce or Eliminate to Meet Her Budget

Cable TV	$80
Defer house maintenance	$75
Cheaper meats and food	$150
Give up restaurants	$150
Minimize new clothes	$150
Cut hair at home	$50
Psychotherapy	$200
Summer camp	$120
Vacations	$250
Total savings	$1,275
Revised budget	$4,350
Available support	$3,900
Persistent deficit	$450

Sara's Perspective

Sara feels guilty about the divorce. She feels sorry for Max but feels that Max should have tried harder during marriage counseling. But she feels most guilty about the children. Everything she has read and learned from her friends is that one should minimize the change the children have to endure. The less change the children have to have, the better for them. She feels very strongly that she and the children should stay in the house and that it is unthinkable that the kids should have to change schools. She understands that money is tight but does not want to go back to work. First of all, the children need her. Who else will take them to after-school music lessons and soccer and gymnastics and tutoring and all the other places three busy kids have to go? Unsupervised kids, particularly teenagers, get into trouble, and Sara is already worried about the erratic tendencies of her middle child. Besides, she no longer has a career. Sixteen years away from the computer business have rendered her skills obsolete. She would need a solid year of retraining, and then the starting position would likely pay only a small salary for years. By the time she got done paying for childcare and housekeeping, she would have almost nothing to show for her efforts. And when she looks at the list of budget cuts she would have to make, she shudders to think what life will be like with none of the amenities the kids are used to. How could she possibly explain that to the kids?

Max's Perspective

Max is against the divorce because he understands what an economic disaster it will be. He is 50 years old, and what will he have to show for his life if he has to give up half of his assets and live on less than half of his income? He has created a budget and figures that he needs at least $4,500 a month if he is to afford a small house of his own and have a place where the kids can spend time with him. Sara is telling him that she needs at least $5,000 a month and that she thinks he should pay it for the benefit of the children. If Sara wants this divorce, she will have to absorb some of the risks and the changes. She can go out and get a job and support herself. She can either move out of the house and let Max stay, or she can sell the house so that both of them can buy small townhouses in the next town. It would be tough on the kids to have to move, but they are strong kids and would manage well. Sara needs to take some responsibility. As it is, Max will have to give up half of his 401K and can say good-bye to retirement. He feels he will never be able to save and is worried about how to send the kids to college.

ECONOMIC ISSUES AND EMOTIONS

We live in society in which the sense of well-being of many people is inextricably related to their ability to consume. I was raised—as were most of my peers—in a house that was at most 1,200 square feet. The average starter home today is about 2,300 square feet, and the number of people who are building houses of 5,000 or 7,000 square feet is growing. Big houses, fancy cars, and even fancier restaurants and vacations have become part of the taken-for-granted reality of the baby boomers and their children. My father regarded a car as a machine to provide transportation from one place to another. Many of my clients regard a car as a garment to be worn as a personal statement. And in the absence of such amenities, my clients feel deprived. Faced with the need to retrench upon divorce, they feel as if they are "going backward." That is, life is regarded as a linear progression toward ever higher levels of consumption and security, and the interruption of that progression becomes a personal as well as an economic crisis. But economic retrenchment is the norm for most divorcing people. Only the wealthy or the very frugal can get through a divorce without major revisions in their consumption patterns. So, the extent to which a client is reluctant to adapt to this reality will define the challenge for the therapist.

As we can see from the case of Max and Sara, the reluctance of each partner to accept the full implications of economic retrenchment sets them up for a legal struggle. Both seek to shift more change and risk to the other, so as to endure less change themselves. And it is very easy to create a justification why the other partner should absorb more change and dislocation, thus reducing the impact on oneself. It's for "the benefit of the children." Or, "It's because it was her idea to divorce that she ought to accept more change." The justifications offered can, at times, be remarkably transparent. I recall one client who needed a new car and actually reported with utmost seriousness that she had researched all cars for their safety record and that it was clear that the children would be safest if she bought a Mercedes Benz. And, of course, the legal system is tailor-made to support clients in their illusions and desires to shift change to their spouses. As was noted in Chapter 6, the adversarial lawyer is trained to get as much as possible for his or her client and to shift disproportionate burdens to the other spouse. The lawyer has no commitment to fairness from the family's perspective but is predisposed to get the best deal for his or her own client. So, the support and encouragement of the lawyer are added to the rationalization of the client. Although there are some lawyers who counsel moderation and provide a reality check, therapists should not assume that their clients have engaged such lawyers.

The challenge for the therapist is twofold. First, the therapist needs to help the client hold him- or herself responsible for accepting a fair measure of change and dislocation without resort to blame, guilt, recrimination, or self-pity. This is the essence of being a grown-up. All the rationalizations that help the client justify focusing on the partner and what the partner should do just delay the inevitable and provoke avoidable conflict. Second, the therapist needs to help the client explore the feelings that are evoked by the realization that less money is going to be available to spend on things that the client believes are necessary to his or her sense of well-being. For some people, the perception of downward economic mobility is experienced as a genuine assault on the self. Many clients will need help in avoiding a retreat into blaming as a way of deflecting the economic realities of divorce. It is not enough to simply validate the client's feelings and empathize with his or her resentment and worry. Such intervention must also set the stage for encouraging the client to accept responsibility and to plan for retrenchment without retreating into belligerence or self-pity.

Clients also need help in accepting that divorce requires changes in the level of consumption of the children. Some psychological literature has promoted the notion that the best way to protect children from the consequences of their parent's divorce is to minimize the changes experienced by the children.[1] According to this viewpoint, children should be able to stay in their home and continue with all the same activities and educational opportunities to which they have become accustomed. If the child is in private school, she should stay there. If he takes piano lessons, he should continue. If she is used to going away to summer camp, she should go. And in an ideal world I would heartily agree with this perspective. Unfortunately, few divorcing couples enjoy the requisite level of wealth to sail blithely on as if nothing has happened. So, here is what often happens. Typically it is the mother who will be the primary residential parent and it is with her that the children will spend 60–70% of their time. So, if the kids are with her and the kids need the house, then she also gets to stay in the house. It is the father who must then move out. But to where shall he move? If the mother makes no major budget cuts (for the benefit of protecting the children), very little of the father's income is left to support his own household. He is told that it is his duty, in the interest of protecting the children, to find a way to manage on whatever is left. Look back at Max and Sara. If the children are to be protected from change, Max must pay Sara $5,600 of his $6,500 take-home pay, leaving him $900 a month on which to live. He simply cannot do it even if he strips his life of every possible amenity. And even after Sara strips her and the children's budget of all the luxuries and discretionary expenses, she still needs $4,300 a month, leaving Max with $2,200 a month to meet all his expenses. It is possible for him to manage a very austere lifestyle on that, but not the middle-class standard to which he is accustomed.

The truth is that for Max and Sara and most middle-class couples, the notion of protecting the children from experiencing signifi-

[1]See Wallerstein, J., & Blakeslee, S. (1990). *Second chances*. New York: Tichnor and Fields.

cant change is a pipedream unless one or both parents are reduced to penury. But if that happens, at least one parent is going to end up depressed and bitter, and I submit that that is very bad for the children. For Max and Sara, life is just too expensive unless Sara goes back to work. But that change can produce a crisis for her. Sara has enjoyed being a homemaker and has developed her identity around that role for 15 years. She does not feel competent to go out into the world to compete, and she worries that her children will not get the required supervision and nurturing if she is away all day at a job. This can make her fearful and angry with Max for not sacrificing enough for the children.

Clients like Sara and Max need help in sorting out the competing needs of the adults and children in the family. This is one of the major challenges of a mediator, but mediators need all the help they can get from therapists who are seeing the clients–either individually or in family therapy–while they are in mediation. As we noted in the Introduction, the concept of the "best interests of the child" must be reframed as "the bests interests of the family." Ultimately, children will do about as well as their parents do in adapting to the divorce. Clients need help in understanding the need for balance and in fully appreciating that they have a vested interest in seeing that their spouse thrives.

CHANGING CAREERS

Changing careers, particularly for mothers who have been homemakers, is an especially emotional issue. Although about 70% of mothers are employed at least part-time, many have long subordinated their careers to raising children. Many have taken years off the jobs altogether, and many others have worked part-time. Still others have limited their vocational choices to such jobs as teaching that left them additional time off to be with their children. Now, in the face of a clear economic necessity, they suddenly have to earn more money. For some, it means acquiring a career for the first time. For others, it means seeking jobs that pay more and are full-time but that leave them less time and energy for their children. Many such women are resistant, because they believe the children will suffer and because they genuinely enjoy and take pride in their roles as mother and housekeeper. In these cases, both men and women need guidance and counseling. I see too many men who begin the divorce with an angry insistence that their wives get first-time jobs or higher-paying jobs in order to bridge the financial gap. Even when these men are correct that this radical change needs to occur, their insistent and undiplomatic stance creates resistance where resistance could be avoided. They need coaching on how to treat the subject so that they do not defeat themselves. They need to resist their impulse to push even though they themselves are feeling anxious.

This is where the discipline of budgets helps. I never tell women that they have to get a job. I require them to prepare their most frugal budget and then to help explain where the money will come from. If your clients are in mediation, the mediator will usually require this exercise. But if they are not yet in mediation, there is no reason that any therapist with even minimal arithmetic skills cannot help clients to do this. It is only when faced with the inability to stretch income to meet an irreducible budget overrun that the woman will herself decide that she has got to increase her income. And it is only when she decides that for herself that she will be motivated to seek the kind of professional help–such as career counseling and help with résumé preparation and interviewing skills–that is needed for a successful job search.

Although changing careers is more often an issue for women, it can often be an issue for men as well. The husband who is a chronic or recent underachiever may feel acute resentment at being left behind by his higher-achieving wife. The most acute example here is the "househusband" who has decided to stay home and perform the homemaking function while his wife has pursued her career. Although a few couples are successful with this role reversal, many others are not. When I see such a couple in mediation, invariably the wife is initiating the divorce because she resents the unproductive husband and has lost respect for him. True sexual equality is still not commonly practiced. These househusbands will need the same kind of encouragement to return to work and develop careers as their female counterparts. And although we see an increasing number of cases in which men receive alimony, this is still a very small part of the divorcing population. Because the majority of men remarry within 2 years of divorce, and because alimony ceases upon remarriage, it is only those men who fail to rebuild their lives who will collect alimony for very long.

"SHOULD WE KEEP THE HOUSE?"

One of the most trying issues for many couples is trying to decide whether they need to sell the marital home. Here is a prime example of economic realities clashing with emotional issues. The impulse to keep the house usually springs from the desire to minimize change for the children. "It's bad enough that their parents are getting divorced. How can we ask them to give up their home too?" Or, "The children are settled in their schools. It's too big a change to move them at this critical time." The children are not the only reason for keeping the house. If it is the mother with whom the children will live, she will often argue that it is too much to ask of her to manage a move at this time. She is overwhelmed with the tasks of adapting to single motherhood, is overwhelmed with the necessity of going back to a full-time job, and is trying to rebuild her social life. "How can you ask me to move, on top of all of that?" Besides the house is *home.* For many people, particularly those who have invested great effort and creativity in decorating the house, the house is not simply a dwelling but also a stage on which the homeowners present themselves to the public. That is, they regard the house as a public statement about them, who they are, what their status is, and their value in the world. For such a person, moving from the house is a particularly great blow, particularly if it involves moving to a smaller or "lesser" house.

Furthermore, a divorcing partner–for example, a husband–may resent the assumption that he has to leave the house and move into an apartment and resent the implication that he will live at a lesser standard of living than his wife. "Why should I have to live in a hole in the wall while she lives in the house I struggled to buy? Let's sell the house and use the money to buy two smaller houses."

Here is where the initiator versus noninitiator distinction again plays a key role. It is the noninitiator who sees only loss coming from the divorce, and because he or she sees no gains, that person struggles to minimize losses. Because the move from the marital home feels like such a major change, it is often the noninitiator who fights the hardest not to move. When men are the noninitiators, the struggle over the house can morph into a custody fight. The house and the children become conceptually fused. "If I am the primary parent and if the children should stay in the house, then I, as primary parent, will stay in the house. Therefore, I should have custody of the children. I am just as good a parent as she is. If she wants a divorce, let her leave, and let her leave the children with me." I have long suspected that the great majority of custody fights involve noninitiating men who are hanging on to the kids as a way to hang on to the house and thus preserve the structure of their lives. But there are strong emotions surrounding the issue of the house itself. However, the decision must ultimately be determined by economic considerations. If the family can afford to keep the house without financially crippling either parent, then it probably should. But if the parents cannot afford it, the house should be sold. So, what are the indicators of affordability? The first issue is cash flow. How large are the mortgage and tax payments relative to the monthly income of the parent in the house?

Let us return briefly to Max and Sara. A reliable rule of thumb is that the housing costs for the mortgage, related taxes, and insurance should not exceed 30% of gross (pretax) income. In fact, this is the most common standard used by mortgage underwriters. If Sara is to stay in the house and not exceed this standard, her monthly mortgage and tax payments require a gross monthly income of $5,800. But Max earns only $80,000 per year. For Sara to keep the house she needs the equivalent of $70,000 a year in pretax income. Obviously, unless she is prepared to return to work and earn about $30,000 a year, she cannot afford to stay, because there is no reasonable circumstance under which she will receive 88% of Max's income. Her best-case hope for support in court is $40,000 a year, about half of Max's income. So, her continuing ability to stay in the house and her imminent return to employment are clearly linked, and the sooner she is helped to realize this, the better. These are mathematical certainties that can be mastered by anyone with access to pencil and paper, and communicated in the therapy office.

There are several other possibilities that sometimes help. Sometimes, but not always, refinancing the house can help lower the monthly cost. If interest rates have dropped significantly, refinancing might lower the cost. If the mortgage is old (15 years or more), refinancing may help. And if the parties have a 15-year amortization, they can often lower the monthly cost by refinancing with a 30-year amortization. This means that the mortgage principal is paid off over 30 years instead of 15 so that the monthly payment is smaller. All these options should be reviewed. But it is the exceptional case in which they will make a major difference. Many couples buy houses that stretch their finances to begin with. I have seen many two-income couples buy a house in which the wife's entire paycheck is devoted to the monthly mortgage payment. For such couples, holding on to the house is simply unrealistic.

The second major financial factor that shapes whether the couple needs to sell the house is how much equity is in the house and what other assets the couple possesses. Let's look once again at Max and Sara. Their home is worth $300,000 and has a mortgage of $180,000. Their equity (value – mortgage = equity) is $120,000. Their only other assets are Max's 401K plan of $140,000 and an IRA of $20,000. Max, who is well into middle age, argues that the equity in the house is, for all practical matters, the only available asset that will allow him to ever buy another house. He will be paying alimony and child support for a long time and will not be able to save money during that time. To cash in the retirement accounts would incur interest and penalties of about 40%, and his accountant has advised him that that would be a very bad idea. So, as long as Sara stays in the house, Max cannot buy a house of his own. He is willing to live that way for a year or two but not for longer than that.

If the couple had significant other assets, the problem would be simpler. Suppose that they also had a stock account worth $150,000. Now there is enough cash available for Max to buy his own house without selling the marital home. Conceivably, if it were sufficiently important, the couple could cash in their retirement accounts, net about $100,000 after taxes and penalties and, at the sacrifice of long-term security, allow Max to buy his house. This can be a very emotional issue, and the couple needs help in sorting out the alternatives and making choices that balance short-term and long-term concerns. What neither of them can afford to do is to dismiss the concerns of the other, and both need encouragement to consider all the alternatives. This is another issue on which the therapist's insistence on a long-term view of the future can bear fruit.

CONCLUSION

Although the division of assets involves much technical information about finance, law, and taxes, therapists cannot afford to be scared off by the technical jargon. Because the division of assets is so fraught with emotional issues that lawyers can only aggravate, the therapist should be closely involved in these discussions with clients. The way the client manages change and loss in the divorce will shape the outcome of the divorce and determine whether the client has a good or bad divorce. The therapist's support and wisdom here can make all the difference to a successful outcome.

13 Wrapping Up the Agreement

At some point in the divorce negotiation, enough agreement has been reached that the time has come to tie up the loose ends, finish the agreement, and have the lawyers draft the final agreement. In this short chapter I want to sensitize the therapist to some of the problems that can arise at this stage and suggest some ways to manage them.

GETTING HUNG UP ON THE DETAILS

For some people the final details can be more difficult than the core agreement. I recall a case I mediated that was rather complex because it involved not just the dissolution of the marriage but also the business partnership the couple had together. After a lengthy and sometimes acrimonious negotiation, the parties had reached agreement on what I thought were all the important points. I drafted a memorandum of understanding reflecting the agreement of the parties. Now it was time for their lawyers to draft the formal agreement.

During the mediation the husband had often demonstrated what might be called an obsessive style of decision making. Even things that I thought were obvious required long periods of reflection, deliberation, and consultation with his lawyer. This pattern of behavior had probably doubled the time it took to mediate the agreement, and I had often had to calm down the wife when she complained about his obsessing over everything. It was his way, I explained, and pressuring him to decide was clearly counterproductive; so, for 4 months I counseled patience. The husband insisted that his lawyer draft the separation agreement. My memorandum was six pages long. I was dumbfounded when after 3 months of delay the husband's lawyer produced a proposed settlement agreement that was 96 pages long. Although some lawyers are more verbose than others, even a verbose lawyer ought to be able to address all the issues in less than 25 pages. But it appeared that my obsessive client had chosen an obsessive lawyer, and together they were prepared to battle over every nuance, every remote contingency that "might happen," and every word. They had also introduced many clauses that were essentially unnecessary but had at every opportunity shaded the wording to slip in small advantages for this client. When the wife's lawyer reviewed the document, I thought he would become apoplectic. He threatened to call off the deal and litigate the matter.

I convinced the parties that it would be a shame if, after all the work and in the presence of a perfectly workable agreement, the parties were to go to war. I convinced the parties and their attorneys to sit with me in mediation and go through the proposed agreement until the details were resolved.

In the first stage of the mediation it had taken 15 hours of work to bring the parties to agreement. Now, in this second stage of mediation, after all the important points had already been agreed, we proceeded to spend 30 more hours mediating the language of the husband's attorney's draft. It was an extremely tedious and trying experience, and I had to work hard to keep the wife and her attorney from walking out. But finally we got it done, and the mediation was over. This case taught me two things. First, the personalities of lawyers can easily defeat an agreement, and clients are seldom aware when it happens. And second, how people respond to details in an agreement can be a product of complex personality and emotional style issues.

Where these issues play out is in the management of risk. Both parties in divorce and their attorneys may try to shift the risk of even remote eventualities to the other side. A common concern, for example, is the fear that one of the parents will decide to move out of the state and take the children, therefore depriving the other parent, typically the father, of routine contact with the children. Undoubtedly, in some cases, the fear is well grounded. The divorcing couple moved to North Carolina from California a year earlier to follow the husband's job, say, and the wife's family, friends, and entire support network was back in California. When the husband decides he wants a divorce, he worries that the wife will want to go home and insists on language to prevent it. But in most cases there is nothing that suggests that the wife has ties elsewhere or has any reason to move. Nevertheless, I have seen husbands insist, at the risk of the agreement, that the wife must agree not to move. In fact, it serves little purpose to put restrictive clauses in the agreement, because the court will ignore them anyhow. But, depending on the style of the husband, this can become a major issue even though the probability is slight that the wife would move.

For the therapist, there is a rich opportunity to help clients maintain realistic perspectives when they try to protect themselves from remote risks. There are cases in which a client, who would otherwise be relaxed about an issue, is goaded into anxiety by a lawyer whose own style is to fight aggressively over every risk, however remote. The therapist can monitor these discussions and challenge the client to weigh the real risks against possible damage to the agreement and the ongoing relationship with the spouse.

SYMBOLIC ISSUES

I recall a case in which we had successfully resolved numerous issues related to children, money, and property. The issues had been complex, and the assets distributed were in the millions of dollars. Although the discussions had frequently been acrimonious, the couple was still able to talk to each other. It also appeared that what had begun as a struggle over custody had been resolved by a cooperative parenting arrangement. Then trouble struck. Sometime before the couple decided to divorce, the husband had purchased a bracelet worth perhaps a thousand dollars as an intended Christmas present for his wife and had kept it in the safe deposit box. The wife was aware that the bracelet was there and wanted it. She was worried that he would give it to his girlfriend and was determined that that would not happen. He was equally determined that the wife not get it and insisted it was his own property. For most of the hour the two wrangled over the bracelet. I observed that it was ironic that after easily distributing millions of dollars they were deadlocking over a thousand-dollar bauble. I suggested that the economic value of the bracelet could not possibly be at issue and that this must be a symbolic issue. The bracelet had come to represent a struggle quite apart from its value, and if the case was to be resolved, we would have to settle the matter symbolically. It wasn't that either wanted the bracelet–it was that each was determined to deny it to the other. So, why not cut it into two pieces and give half to each? They both readily agreed, and the agreement noted that the bracelet was to be taken to a jeweler and cut into two equal pieces. It was only when the agreement was written and ready to be signed that they began to feel foolish and decided to give the bracelet to their infant daughter upon her 16th birthday.

This case is typical of many I have seen in which one or both partners is still ambivalent about the divorce or still has not let go emotionally of the spouse. So, one or both seize on some minor issue and blow it up until it threatens the agreement itself. The issue can involve some aspect of parenting, such as who will do homework with a child, some piece of property, or some minor contingency concerning support. What matters is that a minor issue takes on major proportions because it represents a symbolic struggle rather than a substantive one. Lawyers may or may not catch on and counsel the client to be reasonable. But it depends on the style of the lawyer, and small issues can quickly become deal killers. The therapist here can be the voice of reason and sanity that saves the agreement and avoids a wreck.

DRAFTING THE AGREEMENT

The final document that resolves the divorce and governs the post-divorce life of the parties is called the settlement agreement (see Appendix 13.1 for a sample agreement). It may also be referred to as the property agreement or the divorce agreement. All are the same thing. The document sets forth the details of the couple's agreement on all issues related to children, money, and property. It may also address secondary issues such as life insurance, health insurance, and who gets the tax exemptions for the children. It will also contain a lot of "boilerplate," that is, standard clauses found in every agreement that deal with such matters as the jurisdiction of the court, what happens if a clause is found invalid, and other concerns that arise in all contracts.

Questions may arise about which lawyer is to draft the agreement. If the divorce has been mediated, most mediators prepare a memorandum of understanding that one lawyer will then use as the basis for a draft of the agreement. A few mediators who are experienced divorce lawyers will actually draft the agreement itself for review by the parties' lawyers. If the case has not involved a mediator but has been negotiated directly by the lawyers, they will decide who does the final draft. Ultimately, the agreement will not be signed until both lawyers have approved the language. Generally I have not had much trouble getting the lawyers to agree and finish up the document. But now and then I run into a lawyer who insists on trying to shade every clause so that it shifts various benefits to his or her client to the detriment of the other client. Or, we run into the lawyer who wants to add a clause that deals with every conceivable remote eventuality. When this happens, the case bogs down, and the clients become frustrated.

This is a time when clients have to take control of their lawyers. An intrepid therapist can help the client analyze why the agreement has become endangered. I say intrepid because many therapists may feel intimidated about trying to question the technical judgment of a lawyer. But I do not suggest that the therapist substitute his or her professional judgment for that of the lawyer. Rather, I am suggesting that the therapist support the client in holding the lawyer accountable by asking the lawyer to justify the risks and benefits at issue in the drafting of the agreement. Few divorce agreements are so complex that they should give rise to complicated drafting issues. More often than not, the problem will be a stylistic issue of one of the lawyers, and clients must be proactive in ensuring that they do not pay thousands of dollars struggling over trivial and remote possibilities. Again, the therapist has an opportunity to be the voice of reason.

CONFLICT RESOLUTION

Most mediators recommend that the separation agreement incorporate a clause that requires the couple to return to mediation when a dispute arises that they are unable to resolve themselves. They are required to make a good-faith effort at mediation before either can apply to the court for relief. Of course, if one party requests mediation and the other refuses, the requesting party is then free to go to court. Few lawyers are familiar with such clauses, and some lawyers who are generally hostile to mediation resist them. But if the client insists and both parties agree, the lawyers must include a mediation clause. I strongly suggest them in every case. I have worked with numerous couples that had postdivorce problems and worked them out easily in mediation at a savings of many thousands of dollars. Mediation clauses are a no-lose proposition.

A more progressive clause that can also be added is an arbitration clause. An arbitration clause requires that, if the couple is unable to resolve the dispute, they submit the dispute to binding arbitration rather than go to court. Arbitration is generally cheaper and faster than conventional court processes, and it is being used in divorce with greater frequency. Arbitration decisions are generally not appealable to higher courts, although in states that permit the arbitration of custody issues (most but not all states) the court reserves the right to review the arbitrator's decision.

Whether the couple incorporates a mediation clause alone or a mediation/arbitration clause, the important thing is for them to decide how future disputes will be handled in the least costly and disruptive manner. Therapists should support such measures enthusiastically.

APPENDIX 13.1. SAMPLE SETTLEMENT AGREEMENT

Agreement

Dated this ____ day of ________, 2007, between James Doe, residing at 12 Birch Road, Maplewood, New Jersey, hereafter referred to as the "Husband," and Brenda Doe, residing at 34 Oak Lane, Maplewood, New Jersey, hereafter referred to as the "Wife."

Witnesseth

WHEREAS the parties were lawfully married on January 3, 1988, and,

WHEREAS one child was born to the marriage, Justin, age 14, and,

WHEREAS, by reason of unhappy differences, the parties now desire to live separately and apart, and have no expectations of resuming marital relations; and,

WHEREAS the parties hereto desire to enter into an agreement for the purpose of confirming their separation, making reasonable provision for the support and custody of the unemancipated child of the marriage, and making such other provisions relating to the settlement of Husband's and Wife's financial and property rights, and other rights and obligations growing out of their marriage relation, or otherwise, as are hereinafter contained; and,

WHEREAS the parties hereto have been fully, separately, and independently advised of their legal rights, remedies, privileges, and obligations by counsel of their own selection and have been advised of their respective properties, property rights, incomes, and expectancies, whether real, personal, direct or indirect, vested or contingent, choate or inchoate; and,

WHEREAS the parties have made independent inquiry and investigation with respect to their rights, remedies, privileges, obligations, properties, property rights, incomes, and expectancies, and have been fully informed of the same with respect to his or her spouse, as the case may be; and,

WHEREAS each of the parties has read and fully understands the terms, covenants, conditions, obligations, and provisions of this agreement and believes it to be fair, just, equitable, adequate, and reasonable, and each of them freely and voluntarily, without compulsion or duress, and free from any influences that might impair their judgment, hereby accepts such terms, conditions, and provisions; and,

WHEREAS the parties intend by this agreement to forevermore settle any and all matters between them including, but not limited to, alimony, support, maintenance, equitable distribution, custody, and visitation, and further intend that this agreement shall be incorporated by reference in and survive a judgment of divorce.

NOW, THEREFORE, for and in consideration of the premises and of the promises, covenants, and agreements hereinafter set forth, it is hereby mutually agreed by the parties hereto as follows:

Part A

1. Alimony

a. The Husband shall pay to the Wife as alimony the sum of $3,000 per month. Alimony shall be includable as taxable income to the Wife and excluded as taxable income of the Husband. Alimony shall cease upon the death of either party, the remarriage of the Wife, or the expiration of 12 years, whichever occurs first.
b. Each party shall be solely responsible for providing his or her own health insurance.

2. Custody

a. The parties shall have joint legal custody of the unemancipated child.
b. The Wife shall be the parent of primary residence for the child.
c. Time with the Husband
   i. Alternate weekends from Friday evening to Monday morning.
   ii. Every Thursday night.

iii. Alternate holidays.
iv. Two weeks' vacation each year, to be scheduled by mutual consent of the parties.
v. Such other times as the parties may agree.

d. Cooperation

The parties agree to act cooperatively in implementing all aspects of the arrangements set forth herein. It is the parties' responsibility to share material information with each other and provide access for each other for all events in the child's life inclusive of each party allowing the other to receive notices pertaining to school, camps, doctors, psychologists, or any other mental health provider and shall be kept informed by each other on all matters relating to the child's health, schooling, and activities.

3. Child Support

a. Amount. The Husband shall pay child support to the Wife for the support of the unemancipated child in the amount of $1,000 per month.
b. Health Insurance. The Husband shall maintain medical insurance for the child. Uninsured medical and dental expenses shall be divided equally between the parties.
c. College. The parties agree that the child should attend college if he is intellectually capable and agree to assist the child relative to his or her ability to contribute. This matter shall be further discussed as the child enters the junior year of high school.
d. Life Insurance. Each party shall maintain $200,000 in life insurance for the benefit of the unemancipated child.
e. Emancipation. Child support shall cease upon the emancipation of the child. Emancipation shall occur upon the first happening of any of the following events:
   i. Graduation from high school or reaching age 18, whichever occurs last. However, if the child goes to college directly following graduation from high school, emancipation shall be tolled for a period of 4 consecutive years if the child remains in college for that period. In no event shall child support be paid beyond the child's reaching age 22. Moreover, if the parent paying child support contributes at least one-half of the cost of the child attending college away from home, child support for the child shall be reduced by one-half during the years that the child is attending college.
   ii. Marriage of the child.

iii. Death of the child.
iv. Entry into the military.

f. Modification. Child support shall be subject to renegotiation and review every 2 years to take account of changes in the income of the parties and the Child Support Guidelines of the Courts of New Jersey.

4. Equitable Distribution

a. Marital Home. The marital home shall be sold, and the net proceeds of sale shall be divided equally between the parties.
b. Retirement Funds. The Retirement accounts of the parties shall be equalized by transferring the appropriate amount from the Husband's account to the Wife's account.
c. Bank Accounts. All bank accounts, brokerage accounts, and other securities shall be divided equally between the parties.
d. Automobiles. Each party shall retain his/her own automobile.
e. Household Goods. The household furnishings shall be divided equally between the parties.
f. Miscellaneous Property. Any and all personal property not specifically mentioned in this agreement that is presently in the possession, ownership, or name of the respective party as of the execution of this Agreement will remain in their individual possession and ownership and shall include but not be limited to personal possessions, cars, bank accounts, stocks, bonds, jewelry, and other such property. Any stocks, bonds, or other investments or checking accounts or savings accounts jointly held by the parties as of the execution of this Agreement shall be divided in accordance with the parties' mutual agreement as set forth herein.

5. Dispute Resolution

The parties agree that in the event any dispute arises between them concerning this Agreement, they will attempt good-faith mediation before resorting to court proceedings. They shall choose a mediator acceptable to both parties.

6. Taxes

The parties shall file joint tax returns for the year 2007. They shall share equally in any tax liability or refund. In subsequent years the Wife shall be entitled to claim the tax exemption for the child.

Part B: Other Provisions

1. *Recitals Acknowledged*

All matters stated in the "WHEREAS" clauses set forth on pages 1 through 3 hereof are true and correct, and constitute a part of this Agreement to the same extent as if contained in the body hereof.

2. *Effective Date of This Agreement*

The effective date of this Agreement shall be the latest date of the signing of this Agreement.

3. *No Tax Deficiencies*

Each party represents that there are no tax deficiency proceedings or tax audits currently extant. If there is a deficiency assessment pending against them, or should one arise, each party represents and warrants to the other that he or she has duly paid all income tax, state and federal, and any assessment due on all joint returns filed by the parties. No interest or penalties are due and owing with respect thereto. Each party shall be obligated to immediately notify the other of any notice of audit or tax deficiency or refund upon any joint tax return filed by the parties with any governmental entity.

4. *Future Action for Divorce*

Nothing in this Agreement shall be deemed to prevent either party hereto from maintaining or continuing any action for divorce in any jurisdiction, and, upon request of either party, this Agreement may be entered into evidence and be appended to any judgment of divorce rendered by such court of competent jurisdiction.

5. *Responsibility for Debts*

Subject to the provisions of this Agreement, each party covenants and represents that he or she has not heretofore incurred or contracted, nor will hereafter incur or contract, any debt, charge, or liability whatsoever for which the other may be liable, except as has been previously set forth. Each party covenants that at all times he or she shall keep the other free, harmless, and indemnified of and from any and all debts, charges, or liabilities contracted or incurred by them individually or jointly with the other for which they are or may become liable.

6. *Separate Residence*

The Husband and Wife shall continue to live separate and apart from each other, and each shall be free from interference, authority, and control by the other as fully as if he or she were single and unmarried, and each may conduct, carry on, and engage in any employment, business, or trade that to him or her shall seem advisable, at such place or places as he or she may from time to time choose, for her or his sole or separate use and benefit, free from any control, restriction, or interference, directly or indirectly, by the other party.

7. *No Molestation*

Neither of the parties shall, in any way, molest, trouble, disturb, or interfere with the other in his or her respective peace, comfort, or liberty of action or conduct, and each agrees that they may at all times reside and be in such place and with such relatives, friends, and acquaintances as he or she may choose, whether within or without the State of New Jersey, and each party agrees that he or she will not molest the other, or compel or seek to compel the other party to cohabit or dwell with him or her, or institute or cause to be instituted any action or proceeding for the restoration of conjugal rights, it being mutually agreed that it is, and shall be, lawful for each party at all times hereafter to live separate and apart from the other party.

8. *Law of New Jersey*

This agreement shall be construed and governed in accordance with the laws of the State of New Jersey.

9. *Documents*

The parties agree that they will make available to each other, as and when reasonably required for the purposes of this agreement, various instruments, including but not being limited to various insurance policies (Blue Cross/Blue Shield, Major Medical, homeowner's policy).

10. *Mutual Releases of All Rights in the Estate of the Other*

Each party shall henceforth hold, possess, and enjoy, for his or her sole and separate use and free from interference and control by the other, all of the real and personal estate, choses in action, and other property of which he or she is or, at any time after the date of closing, may be seized or possessed, and each party releases and relinquishes any and all claims and rights that he or she may have had, may now have, or may hereafter acquire to share, in any capacity or to any extent whatsoever, in the estate of the other party upon the latter's death, whether by way of statutory allowance, distribution in intestacy, or election to take against the other party's Will, or to act as executor or administrator of the other party's estate. Without affecting the generality of the foregoing, and by way of amplification and not limitation, each party waives, releases, and bars himself or herself of all right of dower or courtesy, as the case may be, in any real property that either party now has or may hereafter acquire; and each will, upon request, execute good and sufficient releases of dower or courtesy to the other, or to his or her heirs, executors, administrators and assigns, or will join, at the request of the other, in executing any deed or other instruments affecting such real property; provided, however, that nothing herein contained shall in any way constitute a waiver of the right of either party to a full and complete performance of the terms of this Agreement by the other, nor shall anything contained herein prevent either party from instituting an action for divorce and any defenses either may have to any divorce brought by the other. In further amplification of the aforesaid, neither party shall be deemed, pursuant to any provision contained in this Agreement or in any document or instrument referred to herein or related hereto, to be required or otherwise obligated to make provision for the other in his or her Will. The foregoing is intended to and shall also constitute a waiver of any right of election or similar law.

11. *Mutual Release and Discharge of General Claims*

Subject to the provisions of this Agreement, each party has remised, released, and forever discharged, and by these presents does for himself or herself, and his or her heirs, legal representatives, executors, administrators, and assigns, remise, release, and forever discharge the other of and from all causes of action, claims, rights, or demands whatsoever, at law or in equity, or otherwise, that either of the parties hereto ever had, or now has, or may in the future have, against the other, except any or all causes of action for divorce and any defenses either may have to any such divorce brought by the other.

12. *Independent Advice; Full Knowledge*

The parties hereto declare that this Agreement has been agreed upon and is being executed by mutual consent, each of the parties having had the advice of independent counsel, each of the parties agreeing that the provisions contained herein are fair, just, equitable, adequate, and reasonable based upon their free and voluntary evaluation after consulting with independent counsel, without compulsion or duress, and free from any influences that might impair their judgment; and no warranties or representations of any kind or nature whatsoever have been made to either party by the other party, or by or to any person or counsel acting on behalf of either party, as to his or her present or prospective rights, incomes, or expectancies, and that both fully understand the entire purport, intent, and legal effect of this agreement.

13. *Full Disclosure*

The parties hereto acknowledge and agree that each and every aspect of the financial status of the parties has been fully explained to both the Husband and Wife by their respective attorneys, and the parties expressly acknowledge and, to the extent permissible by law, hereby waive and forevermore release and discharge their rights to an equitable distribution pursuant to the authority of a court of competent jurisdiction.

14. *Severability*

In the event any provision of this Agreement should be held to be contrary to or invalid under the law of any country, state, or other jurisdiction, such illegality or invalidity shall not affect in any way any other provision hereof, all of which shall continue and remain in full force and effect in any country, state, or jurisdiction in which such provision is legal and valid.

15. *Further Assurances*

Each of the parties hereto agrees, at the request of the other, to execute, acknowledge, and deliver to the other any and all instruments or documents and to do any and all such acts that may be reasonably necessary to give full force and effect to the purpose and intent of this Agreement.

16. *Notices*

The addresses of the parties for all purposes under this Agreement shall be those addresses of the parties set forth herein above. Each party hereto may at any time and from time to time change his or her address for all purposes under this Agreement, and advise the other party hereto of such new address, by written notice forwarded to the address of the other party set forth herein above. All notices required to be given hereunder by either party to the other shall be in writing addressed to the other party and mailed by registered or certified mail as provided herein with copies to each party's respective attorneys as set forth herein before or as same may be designated from time to time.

17. Waiver or Modification

Any provision by either party of any of the provisions of this Agreement, or any right or rights hereunder, shall not be deemed a continuing waiver and shall not prevent or stop such party from thereafter enforcing such provisions or rights as to the future, and the failure of either party to insist in any one or more instances upon the strict performance of any one or more of the terms or provisions of this agreement by the other party shall not be construed as a waiver or relinquishment for the future of any such terms or provisions, but the same shall continue in full force and effect. No modification or waiver of any of the terms of this Agreement shall be valid unless in writing and executed with the same formality as this Agreement.

18. Entire Agreement

This Agreement is entire and complete and embodies all understandings and agreements of the parties, and no representations, agreements, undertakings, or warranties, of any kind or nature whatsoever, have been made to the other party to induce the making of this agreement, except as expressly set forth in this Agreement, and each of the parties agrees not to assert to the contrary, and that there is no other agreement, oral or written, existing between them. No oral statement or prior written matter extrinsic to this Agreement shall have any force or effect.

19. Binding Effect

This Agreement shall be binding upon, enure to the benefit of, and be enforceable by and against the parties hereto, their heirs at law, next of kin, respective estates, executors, administrators, assigns, and other legal or personal representatives.

20. Discovery

The parties have not engaged in formal discovery, nor have they exchanged Case Information Statements. Both parties acknowledge that they have the right to complete discovery and that they have been advised by their respective attorneys to avail themselves of their rights. However the parties believe they have full knowledge of their financial situation, and they have chosen to execute this agreement as set forth, and they hold their respective attorneys harmless for not taking discovery.

21. Bankruptcy

All obligations for the payment of money by either party to the other as provided by this Agreement shall not be dischargeable in bankruptcy, and the parties acknowledge that the debts created hereby are of such a nature that they are not dischargeable in bankruptcy.

22. Captions

The titles or captions given to the Articles, subarticles, and subsections in this Agreement have been utilized solely for purposes of convenience, and in no event shall any such title, caption, or table of contents be deemed a part of this agreement or interpretive of any of its language or intent.

IN WITNESS WHEREOF, the parties hereto have hereunto set their hands and seals intending to be legally bound hereby the day and year first above written.

Signed, Sealed, and Delivered in the Presence of:

______________________________	______________________________
Witness	James Doe
______________________________	______________________________
Witness	Brenda Doe

STATE OF NEW JERSEY
COUNTY OF ____________________________

BE IT REMEMBERED that on this ____ day of ________, 2007, before me appeared who is personally known to me to be the individual described in or who executed the foregoing instrument and who duly acknowledged that she executed same.

____________________________, ESQ
ATTORNEY, STATE OF NEW JERSEY

DATED: _______

STATE OF NEW JERSEY
COUNTY OF ____________________________

BE IT REMEMBERED that on this ____ day of ________, 2007, appeared before me who is personally known to me to be the individual described in or who executed the foregoing instrument and who personally acknowledged that he executed same.

____________________________, ESQ
ATTORNEY, STATE OF NEW JERSEY

DATED: ________

14 After the Divorce

REBUILDING LIVES AND MANAGING CONFLICT

The job of the therapist is not necessarily over when the settlement agreement is signed. Divorcing people, particularly those with dependent children, still have to relate to each other as they manage the daily details of life. And they have to resolve differences when the inevitable changes that follow divorce require changes in parenting and financial agreements. In this chapter, we will look at the role of the therapist in helping clients navigate the potentially difficult territory of postdivorce conflicts. Additionally, therapists can help clients to successfully build new lives following their divorce.

DIVORCE INFORMS POSTDIVORCE CONFLICT

Some former spouses resolve their differences better than others. If they had a good divorce, they can generally come to resolution better than if they had a bad divorce. But even those who have had good divorces may get into trouble over changes that neither could have anticipated. In either case the therapist will be aware, because these issues are likely to arise in therapy. Therapists may be consulted because children are having problems or because the child and one parent are at odds. Or, a therapist may see a couple in which one of the partners is remarried and tensions between the new spouse and the stepchildren are souring the new marriage.

In most cases the therapist will want to review the nature of the divorce itself, particularly if the client was not in therapy during the divorce. If you worked with the client through the divorce, you will have a good idea how that divorce proceeded. But if the client is new, a thorough history of the divorce may be warranted. There is considerable chance that the new problems are the product of a bad divorce. As we have seen throughout this book, bad divorce leaves couples with:

- Little or no mutual goodwill.
- A continuing emotional struggle.
- An abiding sense of injustice.
- Poor communication.
- No conflict resolution skills and no mediation clause.

The result for such couples is a high probability of continual conflict in court, and such conflict after divorce exacts the same toll in emotional energy and money as it did during the divorce. The therapist is ideally positioned to influence such clients away from continuing litigation and toward mediation and new conflict resolution skills. And if your interventions are successful, you may even help to save the second marriage.

If, on the other hand, the couple has had a good divorce, your interventions may keep the divorce from turning sour after the fact. It is easier to succeed in such cases, because the couple has a greater sense of optimism about being able to work out satisfactory resolutions. If the divorce was done well, couples begin their postdivorce life with:

- A sense of mutual goodwill.
- Enough trust to give each other the benefit of the doubt.
- Closure on their primary emotional issues.
- A sense that the settlement was fair.
- Communication adequate to cooperative parenting.
- Conflict resolution skills and a mediation clause.

TAKING A HISTORY

If the client was not seen by the therapist during the divorce, a history of the divorce itself should be secured in addition to whatever history is typically taken. The following information may be useful:

- Who was the initiator of the divorce?
- What was the level of conflict during the divorce?
- Was the divorce settled prior to trial, or did it go to trial?

- How much time passed between the initiation of the divorce and its resolution?
- How large were the legal fees? Did the legal fees have a substantial impact on the family finances?
- What has been the nature of the communication between the former spouses since the divorce?
- Are either or both former spouses remarried or with a long-term partner? How have the children adjusted to new partners? What is the relationship between the new partners and former spouses?
- How have conflicts been managed since the divorce?
- What are the immediate issues and problems?

WHAT DIVORCED PEOPLE FIGHT ABOUT

Divorced people fight about children and money. Some of these fights are the result of one of the parties not living up to the agreement. He is supposed to pay $200-a-week child support, and he only pays $100. Or, he pays on the 15th of the month when he had agreed to pay on the 1st day of each month. Or, he arrives to pick up the children, and she tells him they have other plans and will not be coming. People can find endless ways to sabotage their agreements. But when this is what you see, you have to ask "Why?" Is one of them reneging on the agreement simply to be arbitrary and disagreeable? Has one of them found that certain provisions of the agreement are just so onerous that he or she cannot live with them? Or, has something changed that makes it unreasonable to ask that the agreement be enforced as originally agreed?

Some of the fights are about new issues not anticipated by the agreement. She remarries, and the new husband wants to accept a promotion that requires a transfer to another state. This would require that the parenting pattern be renegotiated, and the father is resistant. He remarries, and the oldest daughter takes a dislike to his new wife and refuses to go to her father's house when the wife is present. The 15-year-old son decides that he no longer wants to live with his mother and, over his mother's objection, wants to live with his father. All of these are the inevitable consequences of the changes that follow divorce.

When faced with such problems, former spouses have two options. They can attempt to enforce the agreement as is. Or, they can renegotiate parts of the agreement in an attempt to find common ground. They actually have a third option, which is to live in perpetual noncompliance. But this is such a wretched state of affairs that I do not regard it as an option.

ENFORCING THE AGREEMENT

As a general rule, courts enforce the terms of divorce agreements unless the court finds that the agreement was unconscionable at the onset or unless the court finds that the situation has changed so significantly that it would be unfair to enforce the agreement as originally negotiated. Findings of unconscionability seldom occur in courts. The court must find that the contract is so unfair and one-sided as to be shocking. The client who is simply dissatisfied with the deal after the contract has been signed will not find much relief in court. Courts, however, will throw out an agreement if it is found that one of the parties engaged in fraud or if one of the parties can prove that he or she signed the agreement without understanding it or as a result of duress. But these are unusual events. Chances are strong that the court will order the agreement enforced as negotiated. So, does this mean that if your client believes that his or her former spouse is violating the agreement he or she should just go to court?

RENEGOTIATION

Sometimes we win the battle but lose the war. Enforcing an unfair agreement only breeds a greater sense of resentment and leaves the defeated party ever more vigilant for opportunities to get even. If your client's spouse is in violation of the agreement, the client should nevertheless seek mediation before resorting to the courts. If the original divorce was resolved in mediation, the agreement probably contains a mediation clause, so both are obligated to try mediation. And if the divorce was resolved in a conventional adversarial negotiation, it will be unlikely to have a mediation clause. So, here is an opportunity to try mediation and to get the divorce out of the adversarial system.

By suggesting mediation to the spouse, the client accomplishes two things. First, the client provides a demonstration of intent to pursue the matter and seriousness about resolving the issue. Second, the client demonstrates a willingness to listen and, perhaps, even agree to modification to make the agreement less onerous to the former spouse. Divorce agreements, like all complex human endeavors, are subject to error. Perhaps the other spouse made concessions out of fear of a trial, fear of being humiliated, or out of guilt or a sense of intimidation. Perhaps the lawyer representing the other spouse was an ineffective negotiator or the former spouse was confused about the implications of some aspect of the agreement. Maybe this is a bad or unfair agreement. If any of those things are possible, the client should at least be willing to look at the agreement anew. It may be an opportunity to establish some new principles of cooperation and respect that could change the tone of the postdivorce relationship. An abiding sense of injustice sours and poisons relationships forever. Mediation is an opportunity to address not just the specific issue of noncompliance but also the sour relationship itself. Bad agreements can usually be fixed, and the effort is well spent.

CHANGES OF CIRCUMSTANCES

Most court battles in the years following divorce are related to the inability of the parties to come to agreement when changes in life's circumstances require changes in the arrangements for children and money. With respect to money, the changes usually involve the attempt by one party to increase or decrease alimony or child support. The attempted change is premised on the fact that one or the other's income has significantly changed, thereby compelling increased or decreased support. We will discuss this shortly, but first we will look at changes in circumstances that affect children.

The issues of change affecting children include changes in the custody and visitation arrangements. It may be as minor as adjusting the visitation schedule to accommodate business travel or plans of the children. Or, it may involve an adolescent's request to no longer move between two households. More difficult are proposed changes in the basic parenting arrangement, in which one parent–typically the nonresidential parent–is seeking to have the child live principally with him or her. And the most difficult of all are "removal" cases in which one parent is moving far away and wants to take the child along.

States laws differ on these issues. In all states the court retains jurisdiction at all times. This means that, no matter what is in the agreement, the court retains the right to change the arrangement when so required by the "best interests of the child." It is always possible for a former spouse to seek a change in the parenting agreement. But when changes involving the children are resolved in court, the litigation can sour not only the postdivorce relationship between the ex-spouses but can also create havoc between parent and child. Consider the case of Bonnie and Ed.

CASE STUDY: BONNIE AND ED

Bonnie and Ed have been divorced for 6 years, during which time the parties' children, Sarah, age 13, and Tommy, age 11, have lived primarily with Bonnie. They have spent alternate weekends with their dad and have joined him for dinner one evening a week. They enjoy his company because he is funny and easygoing and not much of a disciplinarian. In fact, Bonnie thinks he lets them get away with "murder" and has long been critical of the fact that when they come home from a weekend with Ed it takes her days to get them back in order.

Six months ago Bonnie remarried. Her new husband Will has two children of his own who spend alternate weekends with him. Sarah and Tommy both resent having to share their home and mother with Will's children and find their new stepsiblings whiny and disagreeable. They are also not happy with Will, whom they find bossy, and feel that they do not need yet another tough parent figure in their lives. Ever since Will moved in, the children have been complaining to Ed. Sarah has told her dad that she wants to come live with him to get out of having to cope with the new situation. Similarly, Tommy has told his dad that if Sarah changes homes he wants to change too.

Although this case is based on a real couple, I will provide two alternate scenarios of what happens next.

Scenario 1: Seeking Help from the Lawyer

Ed contacts his lawyer to tell him that his kids are miserable living with Bonnie and Will and that he wants to seek a change in custody. He reports all the resentment felt by the children and tells his lawyer that Sarah's grades have dropped as a result of the new situation and that he fears for the children's welfare if they have to stay with Bonnie. His lawyer writes a letter to Bonnie, who is shocked and outraged by the lawyer's comments that the children would be better served by a change in custody. She regards the problems with the children as a normal problem of transition and is confident everyone will settle down in a year or so. She is angry that Ed communicated through his lawyer instead of talking to her directly and takes this as further evidence that Ed is irresponsible.

Bonnie calls her lawyer and faxes the letter to her. Her lawyer tells her that Ed can indeed seek custody and that if he did, the judge would probably interview the kids and be at least influenced by the children's preferences. She tells Bonnie that the children are old enough that their preference carried some weight with the court but that the judge was not bound by what the children said. Bonnie also learned that, if custody were to be changed, not only would Ed stop paying child support but also might well receive child support from her. She is now furious and believes that this is just Ed's way of seeking a financial advantage.

Bonnie asks her lawyer to respond to Ed's lawyer and tell him that under no circumstances would she agree to such a change. She also calls Ed and tells him off. They end up in a screaming match. Bonnie then confronts Sarah and tells her how disappointed she is in her behavior. She accuses Sarah of making trouble just because she thinks her father will let her get away with anything she wants to do. They also have a shouting match, and Sarah stalks out of the room. The couple is soon locked in litigation.

Scenario 2: Consulting a Psychologist

After several conversations with the children, who tell him they want to change, Ed calls Bonnie. He tells her about his conversations with Tommy and Sarah. He also tells her that he thinks it would be a good idea for the children to come live with him. Bonnie completely disagrees with what he says and tells him that the children are experiencing the ordinary problems of transition and that she believes everything will work itself out. Ed still disagrees. Bonnie suggests that the two consult a child psychologist. Ed, who is skeptical about psychotherapists, reluctantly agrees and says that he will listen but not feel bound by what the psychologist says. At the psychologist's office the two continue their disagreement. The psychologist says that she will need to interview the children but, in her experience, the children would be better served by cooperation between their parents. She says this is more important than who the children live with. She also says that the couple should have a consultation with a mediator and see if they can negotiate a resolution. She promises to see the children if it becomes necessary but advises Ed and Bonnie to try mediation first. The couple agrees.

Comparing the two scenarios offers a clear vision for the potential role and contribution of the therapist. Here the therapist is able to point out the relative costs and consequences of the conflict and to help both parents normalize the behavior and desires of the adolescent daughter. The couple that does not get such guidance ends up in lawyer-dominated conflict. The couple who seek the therapist's help are successfully directed to a more constructive alternative.

Scenario 1: Litigation

Bonnie and Ed litigated the issue for 4 months. During this time the court ordered a custody evaluation, including a home study by a county social worker, a psychological evaluation of both parents and children by a court-appointed custody expert, and an interview of the children by the judge himself. At the hearing both the social worker and the psychologist testified that the children would probably settle down if they stayed with Bonnie but that they would also do well with Ed. The judge, who had been impressed by Sarah's impassioned plea that she be allowed to live with her father, ordered that custody be changed and that the children live with Ed. They were to spend alternate weekends with Bonnie. Ed was to be paid modest child support by Bonnie.

Scenario 2: Mediation

Ed and Bonnie went to see a mediator suggested by the psychologist. The mediator provided each with an opportunity to express his or her views without interruption and made sure that each was heard by the other. He acknowledged that each had legitimate concerns but also confirmed that their only reasonable solution was a cooperative one. In this safe environment Bonnie was able to acknowledge that the tension with Sarah was very difficult for her and that she feared that Sarah was being helped to express normal adolescent rebellion in a particularly destructive manner. She also told how the difficulty with Sarah was straining her relationship with Will and that she would welcome help. She also told Ed that she felt attacked by him and that she felt she was being accused of being a bad mother.

Ed told Bonnie and the mediator that it was very difficult for him to listen to Sarah's complaints and not do anything to come to her rescue. He acknowledged that he had fears about being supplanted by Will in his role as father. He said that he would welcome the opportunity to have the kids full-time, because he missed having more time with them. And he assured Bonnie that he was not motivated by economics and had no interest in having her pay him child support.

After four sessions with the mediator, Bonnie and Ed agreed to some changes to take the pressure off of everyone. They decided that the children would spend more time with their father. Weekends with Ed were expanded from Friday and Saturday nights to Friday, Saturday, and Sunday nights. Additionally the children would spend every Monday overnight with Ed and would spend one continuous month with him during the summer. Child support was left unchanged. Both Ed and Bonnie were pleased with the new arrangement. Ed was pleased to have more time with his kids and felt that he was helping the children cope with their new situation. Bonnie was pleased to have more time with Will undistracted by Sarah's teenage sulking. And she felt relieved that her role as a mother wasn't being attacked. Finally, both felt optimistic that they would be able to work out problems in the future. In fact, they made an appointment to return to mediation in 6 months for one session just to review how things were going.

This mediation here might even have been done by the therapist if he or she felt comfortable. The role of the mediator was to facilitate the communication of the feelings of the parents, normalize the behaviors involved, and help the parties work out a solution that avoided bitterness while permitting necessary adaptation to change. I suspect that the strategy of most mediators and most therapists in such a situation is not dramatically different.

Scenario 1: Postscript

Sarah moved in with Ed. Bonnie was bitter and barely speaking to Sarah. Things between them deteriorated to the point where Sarah simply refused to go to her mother's house. Tommy also went but felt uncomfortable because he worried that he had somehow betrayed his mother. Things were now tense between Will and Bonnie, and they fought over how to pay off the $20,000 in professional fees that had been incurred. The loss of child support and the requirement that Bonnie pay child support to Ed added to her strain.

Nor did Ed escape unscathed. Dealing with Sarah was one thing when she came every other weekend but was quite another now that she was there full-time. She was messy and disorderly, and when he attempted to confront her she was rude and sulky. Living full-time with his teenage daughter turned out to be much more difficult than he had thought. Tommy seemed to be doing OK but often seemed moody and distant. Ed had started a relationship with Cindy, a woman he met at work. But Cindy was unwilling to take on the job of full-time stepmother to a rude teenager and wanted to defer any talk of marriage until Sarah graduated from high school and left for college. Sometimes Ed wondered whether he had done the right thing.

Scenario 2: Postscript

A year later Ed and Bonnie and their children are doing well. The extra time the children spend with Ed has taken the pressure off everyone. Bonnie and Will are getting along and gradually adjusting to their roles as stepparents. There are fewer outbursts between Sarah and her mother, but Bonnie still regards Sarah as a "handful." The children welcome the extra time with their father but wonder why he has become more demanding now that they are at his house more often. And they also wonder how it will work out after Ed and Cindy get married next summer.

COMMENTARY: This story illustrates the choices almost all couples can make when faced with postdivorce conflict about children. It is in their mutual interest to help their children adapt to change. This includes helping the children adapt to change in each other's household without disrupting that household. Each may need help to check the impulse to rescue the child from the other parent unless it is absolutely clear that unalterable harm is coming to that child. As their therapist, you can help them maintain an even keel.

REMOVAL CASES

The most difficult cases I have mediated are divorces in which one parent, the residential parent, decides to move to another state and the distance is so great as to make routine access impossible for the other parent. These are difficult cases because there is so little common ground. The parent who wants to move is seeking a better life. She has been offered a great job in another state or is being transferred because her employer is relocating. Or, her new husband is being transferred and promoted in another state. Or, she wants to return to the place where she grew up in order to have the support of family and friends. To be unable to take the children with her may be a great hardship, because she has to give up an important life opportunity.

But these cases are also heart-wrenching for the other parent, typically the father. It was hard enough giving up daily contact with the kids. Now he is asked to meet his needs as a parent during the summer and holiday vacations exclusively. Why should he have to sustain such a loss? If she wants to go, she can go–but leave the children here. No matter what the outcome, this family is going to experience some painful changes. If ever there was a time to treat each other with grace, this is it.

Because this is such a mobile society, courts have had to deal with an increasing number of such cases. Not only does the law differ from state to state, it also changes over time within many states. For some time in a state the trend may be toward giving the residential parent more leeway by placing the burden of proof on the other parent to prove that the children will be harmed by the move; then the law in that state evolves to place more of a burden on the residential parent and less on the nonresidential parent. Most courts require that the parent seeking the change show a genuine benefit accruing to her (or him) from such a change. They also require a showing that the move will not harm the children or do irretrievable harm to the children's relationship with the other parent. But generally courts seem to be moving in the direction of being more liberal in permitting mothers to move with the children. This is this something that can be guarded against in the original separation agreement. But, even if the mother were to agree to a clause restricting her right to move, courts would be reluctant to enforce any clause that takes away the court's ultimate authority to determine what is in the best interests of the children.

Because these are such difficult situations, no one can provide blanket advice on whether your client should or should not agree to such a move. These must be decided on a case-by-case basis. But there are some things that I tell my clients.

For the residential parent seeking the move:

- Do not deceive yourself. The move will cause considerable pain to your former spouse and should be considered only if you truly have no practical alternative.
- When you propose the move, you should also be prepared to have the children spend most if not all vacation time with the other parent. This means not only that you spend less vacation time with them but also that you need to compensate your ex-spouse wherever possible for the move in other ways.
- Be prepared to share the cost of back-and-forth transportation for the children. It is one of the ways you can demonstrate your willingness to be fair.
- Do not try to justify the move by attacking the other's parenting as a way of minimizing the loss. It does not help to tell the other parent that he was not spending that much time with the kids anyhow.
- Give the other parent as much advance notice as possible and be patient while he reacts. Few parents will take this news with calm indifference.
- Suggest mediation.

For the nonresidential parent:

- It is difficult to win these cases in court. To litigate and lose leaves you in a weakened position to negotiate. It also leaves the two of you embittered.
- If the child spends all summer—about 10 weeks—and two week-long vacations during the school year, that totals 80–90 nights, or about 25% of the time. If you supplement this with one long weekend a month in which you either go to them or they come to you, that adds another 20–30 nights, bringing the total to between 100 and 130 nights per year. This is 30–35% of the total available time. This is more than sufficient for you to retain a robust and full relationship with your children.
- Videophones and computer Internet video setups are inexpensive nowadays. You can talk to and see your children every day. Be creative.
- Suggest mediation.

CHANGES IN FINANCIAL CIRCUMSTANCE

Many postjudgment conflicts concern the modification of support provisions when one or both parties have a significant change in income. In these disputes, the recipient of support seeks an increase if he or she thinks the payer's income has increased or sometimes if her income has decreased. The payer is seeking a decrease in support obligations if he or she thinks the recipient's needs have decreased or if his income has decreased. There are specific laws that apply to how the courts manage these issues, but some general principles apply.

First, the court never gives up its jurisdiction over child support; so, it can change it upon a finding that such a change is warranted. And because child support is the right of the child, the right to seek child support cannot be waived in negotiation. Second, all states now have mandatory child support guidelines that establish some scheme for allocating support obligations between the parents. More often than not, courts will fall back on those guidelines to determine how support will be adjusted in response to changes in circumstances. In the typical divorce where the father is paying child support, courts will increase the support if the father's income increases substantially. The general sense of the law is that children are entitled to share in the good fortune of their parents. So, if his income has increased by half, you can be fairly certain that child support is going to increase. Similarly, if his income drops significantly, child support will probably be decreased until his income is restored.

In the modern economy many people have volatile incomes. Many employees receive annual bonuses that fluctuate significantly. Many self-employed people have large changes from year to year. If this applies to your client or his former spouse, it is best to have some negotiated formula that automatically applies from year to year.

CHANGING NEEDS OF CHILDREN

Disputes about child support modification sometimes have nothing to do with changes in income but rather concern changing needs or desires of a child. Jeremy is doing poorly in school, and his mother wants him to go to private school, where he can get more individual attention. She seeks additional support from Jeremy's father, who says he cannot afford it and, besides, it's unnecessary. Hailey has been taking ballet lessons for 3 years, and her teacher reports that Hailey is so talented that she should be taking special and expensive lessons. Hailey wants the lessons, and her mother wants the father to pay. He refuses. James has just obtained a driver's license, and his father, with whom he lives, wants James's mother to contribute to the staggering increase in his auto insurance premium. She refuses.

In my experience many of these disputes are not just about money but reflect the failure of parents to work out cooperative parenting arrangements. The distribution of scarce resources between children and their parents is a tricky issue in intact families. It is even more difficult in divorced families. One parent may be more inclined to indulge a child than is another. Or what one regards as a necessity the other regards as a luxury. A danger of these disagreements is the tendency of one parent to inform the child that he or she could have something he or she wants except that the other parent will not help pay for it. If unchecked, this behavior alienates the child from the other parent and harms all family relationships.

When your client presents such problems in therapy, it would be ideal if you can see both former spouses, if you have already worked with both of them. If only one party is your client, then refer the couple to someone else who can see both of them. The dispute over spending on children has emotional roots best explored by a skilled therapist. If the problem cannot be resolved in couple therapy, it should be sent to mediation.

If the original support agreement was negotiated fairly, the agreement will provide that decisions on extraordinary extra expenditures should be made by both parents. Each should have the right to say "no" and should not be criticized if other needs must take priority. Parents trying to do the best for their children can unwittingly get into a situation where children have the opportunity to manipulate one parent through the other. Private schools, expensive summer programs, elective plastic surgery, and expensive lessons are all nice if one can afford them, but most people cannot. Nothing prevents a parent from choosing to indulge a child once in a while, but that parent should not expect the other parent to pay half. Each has a right to a life, and beyond basic support obligations neither has abdicated the right to make parental decisions about spending.

ALIMONY AND CHANGES IN FINANCIAL CIRCUMSTANCES

Alimony is usually based on the standard of living enjoyed during the marriage. Accordingly, recipients of alimony (mostly women) are not entitled to an automatic share of any major increase in a former spouse's income in the way that children are. If the historical income of a husband has averaged $100,000 over the last 5 years of the marriage, and the wife's alimony was based on that income level, the wife is probably not entitled to an increase in alimony if the husband's income doubles as a result of a major promotion that occurs well after the divorce is over. She is probably entitled to an increase in child support—but not alimony. That is because courts hold that children are entitled to share in the newfound fortunes of a parent but alimony is based on the standard of living enjoyed *during* the marriage. On the other hand, a large decrease in the husband's income will usually entitle him to a reduction in alimony, at least until his income recovers. It may seem unfair, but alimony rules are difficult to change.

Reductions in the payer's income and increases in the recipient's income are the most frequent causes of postdivorce disputes. Ideally, these are topics that would be addressed in the original agreement. There are formulas that can be applied to measure the impact of a wife's increasing income on alimony. For example, one couple I worked with recently agreed that for every $2 the wife earned in excess of $30,000 a year, the husband would be entitled to a decrease in alimony of $1. This meant that both would share the benefit of the wife's improving ability to support herself. Remember, in most states alimony is based on need. And in a society in which most women are employed outside the home, there is a powerful supposition that women who can support themselves should do so.

Changes in financial circumstances should be the subject of negotiation rather than litigation. If the couple negotiated well in the original agreement, they should be able to manage these changes as well. If the original agreement was flawed or was poorly negotiated, they need to get to work now and fix it. They should use mediation to negotiate general principles that put an end to the disputes, rather than just waiting for the next outbreak.

IMPACT OF POSTDIVORCE CONFLICT ON SECOND MARRIAGES

The role of therapists in monitoring and resolving postdivorce disputes can often save the second marriage of a client. When people engage in chronic conflict with ex-spouses, it usually has a corrosive effect on their second marriage. Second wives can be resentful of the support being paid to the first wife and pressure the husband to fight his ex. I have seen cases in which the second wife is put in charge of running the litigation against the first wife, or in which the second husband directs the litigation against the first husband. When this occurs, it suffuses the new relationship in the anger of the first and creates innumerable problems. Only the therapist can press clients to analyze how the failed first marriage and the new marriage are beginning to interact in a damaging manner. Stepfamily relationships are difficult, at best. But when the stepparent becomes the prime mover in conflict with the biological parent, the impact on the children is severe. Stepparents should be counseled to let the biological parent deal with the former spouse and to understand the tremendous conflict that can result in pressing a spouse to fight a former spouse. Being a stepparent is daunting under any circumstance, but it is only made worse by ongoing conflict between the former spouses.

CONCLUSION

Good divorces are usually characterized by low levels of conflict between former spouses. Because they both accept change and are able to wish each other well, they are less likely to sabotage each other as each moves on with life. Accordingly, when we see couples with a high level of postdivorce conflict, we usually discover that they had a bad divorce. That is, it was accompanied by a high level of conflict from the beginning, a large role for lawyers, much contact with the judicial system, and great financial and emotional expense. Instead of leaving the couple with a good chance to rebuild, the bad divorce has actually diminished their chances of successful adaptation, and their own lack of cooperation emotionally injures the children, who in turn ruin their parents' lives.

Therapists who see one or both former partners in such high-conflict situations face a daunting task in trying to help the clients understand how the nature of the divorce itself shaped the present state of affairs. In some but certainly not all such cases, a therapist may succeed in helping the couple change the way they relate to each other. Collaboration between therapists and mediators is very useful in these cases, because the unresolved anger of the clients may be more effectively addressed by the therapist while the mediator helps develop alternative agreements that work for the couple.

Concluding Thoughts

A central premise of this book is that a good divorce is not an accident. Bad divorces are often the product of unintentional blundering on the part of clients, their lawyers, and their friends, who fail to understand what is required for a peaceful divorce and overestimate the usefulness of aggressive adversarial behavior. So, bad divorces are usually accidental, in that they produce unintentional injuries that prudence might have avoided. A good divorce can be achieved by couples who intentionally manage their emotions and resources to avoid the common pitfalls of contemporary divorce. This, in turn, requires that those couples become educated quickly in a curriculum that includes:

- An understanding of the emotional process they are experiencing.
- An understanding of the legal process they are experiencing.
- An understanding of the powerful feelings that can lead them astray.
- An understanding of the ways to manage strong feelings and pursue legitimate interests.
- An understanding about how the emotional choices they make will interact with the legal decisions they will make.

A good divorce also requires those couples to master certain skills that include:

- The ability to negotiate with each other until viable agreements are reached.
- The ability to prepare and manage budgets as a way of getting control over financial management issues.

- The ability to master collegial communication as a replacement for the intimate communication they have shared in the past.
- The ability to manage their strong feelings that can get in the way of constructive action.

As clients increase their understanding and skills in these directions, the chances that they will achieve a good divorce increase. So, the question we ask is: Who is going to provide couples with the teaching, guidance, and leadership needed to acquire the requisite skills and understanding? We have explored the sources commonly available to divorcing couples. First, couples receive lots of unsolicited advice from friends and relatives, many of whom have themselves experienced divorces. That advice is almost uniformly bad in that it promotes fighting and assumes that divorce is necessarily a war of attrition. Such amateur advisors commonly urge the hiring of aggressive lawyers and beating the other spouse to the punch by raiding bank accounts and cutting off credit cards; moreover, they press their assumptions that the other spouse will engage in tricky maneuvers to hide assets and cheat in the divorce. The collective paranoia urged by this "Greek chorus" does nothing but heighten fear and anxiety and promote fighting between the two parties.

The second source of information is the professionals who consult, represent, and treat divorcing people. They consist primarily of lawyers, with some role played by mental health professionals and financial professionals such as financial planners and accountants. Most of the financial professionals who engage in divorce support are enthusiastic participants in an adversarial process and are primarily motivated to help their clients get as much money as possible without reference to fairness, the impact on the other spouse, or the consequences for family dynamics. I have found few accountants or financial planners who promote peaceful divorce and approach a family's finances from the perspective of "How do we organize this so that everyone thrives?"

Then we have the lawyers, whose culture and assumptions we have discussed at length. There are some lawyers who do a good job of educating clients in the prerequisites of a good divorce, but there are few lawyers who have a solid understanding of the interaction of emotional and legal processes. In my experience, most lawyers inadvertently promote client behavior that causes the relationship between the spouses to deteriorate unnecessarily. Few lawyers have a deep grounding in psychology or philosophy. Few lawyers have specific training in negotiation or communication skills. And the legal culture that emphasizes the representation of the client by the lawyer takes little note of the client's need for growth and autonomy during the process of divorce. So, when we review the skills and understandings established above as requisites to a good divorce, only lucky clients will find lawyers who will provide the teaching, leadership, and wisdom required.

So, where does that leave us? One fact that is important is the role of mental health professionals in supporting the divorce mediation movement over the past 25 years. During that time, divorce mediation has been the most powerful and positive impetus for change in the way people get divorced. And it is from mental health professionals that most of the divorce mediation referrals have come. For many years, other professions provided rigorous resistance to divorce mediation. For the first 10 years of the movement, the divorce legal establishment could best be described as apoplectic. Accountants were mostly negative or, at best, neutral. So, it was to social workers, psychologists, and counselors of many types that those of us who were the earliest practitioners turned to for support and referrals. For the most part, therapists "got it"—and did so quickly. I would estimate that 80% of referrals during the early years of my practice came from mental health practitioners. From that experience, I have become increasingly optimistic that these practitioners could play a larger role in helping couples achieve amicable, constructive, and good divorces.

At the heart of the skills and understanding required for a good divorce is the client's awareness of his or her feelings and how those feelings interact with the surrounding world. All of the powerful feelings associated with divorce—loss, betrayal, fear, loneliness, anger, jealousy, and the like—can drive the client to act in a way that assures a bad divorce. Only the client who is aware of what she (or he) feels, is aware of the choices she has in how to act on those fears, and is aware of the negative consequences of acting out can choose to manage her feelings and act on her interests. And the professional who is most likely to help the client become aware and choose wisely is the therapist.

I am acutely aware that this call to arms for therapists may grate on the sensitivities of some therapists. In conversations about this book with many therapists, responses have varied from very enthusiastic to very skeptical. The abiding—and unfounded—fear of litigation looms large for some, and a general sense of intimidation by the mystique of the legal profession is present in others. Some therapists argue that the interventions suggested here go beyond the proper scope of therapy as they understand it. And I would not presume to get in the middle of complex and contradictory debates over what therapy is and what it is not. But, notwithstanding that endless debate, certain facts remain. You, the therapist, are superbly positioned to prevent a lot of grief, turmoil, and damage to the emotional well-being of your clients and their families. You have the opportunity and the credibility to speak to the emotional choices that face your clients when confronted by divorce. You have the ability to exercise the leadership necessary to direct the client toward acquisition of the knowledge and skills that are the prerequisites for a good divorce. You have the knowledge to teach most if not all of that material. And you have the skills to help the client understand the emotional consequences of the legal strategic and tactical decisions made by the clients and their lawyers. I think that whatever you call it—therapy, coaching, teaching, leading—is immaterial. What is critical is that you do it.

Divorce is about change and transition. With the exception of short childless marriages, divorce requires dramatic and life-changing transitions from every member of the family: changes in parental arrangements, changes in living arrangements, changes in identity, reorganization of social lives, and changes that affect the extended family and former in-laws. The sheer volume of changes can be overwhelming, and they can occur over a long time—up to 5 or more years for many. These changes are scary and can challenge the very psychological structure and coping capacity of all the parties involved while triggering a series of emotional crises. So, while divorce is doubtless a legal process, it is even more certainly an emotional process that should call forth the help of those mental health professionals who are uniquely situated to reduce the trauma of individuals and families. I hope that this book will help more therapists answer that call.

Index